Is Your C

Killing

A healthier you in as little as 8 minutes a day

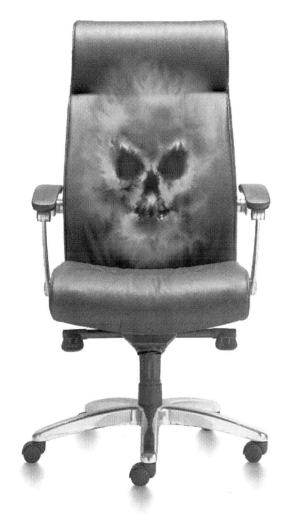

Kent Burden

Is Your Chair Killing You?
A healthier you in as little as 8 minutes a day
By Kent Burden

Copyright ©2012 by Kent Burden

Editor: Jessica Sarra

Cover Art: Heather Montano

Published 2012 by MLF Press, a subsidiary of My Life Fitness, LLC

ISBN: 978-1475236286

IS YOUR CHAIR KILLING YOU?

Kent Burden

TABLE OF CONTENTS

Acknowledgements

I have relied on the wisdom and talents of many people as I crafted this book, but several really stand out. First and foremost I would like to thank my beautiful wife Maria, who listened patiently (and probably feigned interest) as I droned on and on about statistics and anthropology. She allowed me to invade her privacy and journal her every movement for several weeks then let me put it on display for my readers to see. She put up with being blindfolded while working through the movements as I read her the descriptions so the movements made sense. She fixed my lousy punctuation and terrible grammar. Without her this book would never have happened.

I would also like to thank Maria Masters who wrote the article in *Men's Health* magazine that lit the fuse in me about this subject. Her writing enthralled me and made me think, which is what great writing always does.

I am in awe of both Dr. James A Levine and Marc Hamilton, PhD as the leaders in this research here in America. It is their brilliance that lights the way to better health for all.

A big shoutout goes to my editor Jessica Sarra who makes me look like a much better writer than I actually am. (She would hate that I'm using the term shoutout, by the way). I would like to thank Nate Vereb for his can-do attitude and for helping me draw my concept for the cover art from my peanut-sized brain onto paper. I am grateful to Heather Montano for doing the heavy lifting with her remarkable artistic talent to bring the final cover art to life.

They all deserve a standing ovation...and after the ovation, let's keep standing, shall we?

Introduction

Is Your Chair Killing You?

You may not want to sit down, because what I'm about to tell you will shock you. In fact, what I'm about to tell you may rock you to your very core. But whatever you do, don't sit down. The truth is: most of us sit way too much, and all that sitting may be killing you. That's right, killing you! I know what you're thinking: "This guy is a being dramatic." But according to some groundbreaking new research, this statement isn't hyperbole at all. Sitting for long periods of time may be just as bad for you as smoking cigarettes. Now, unless you've been living under a rock for the past ten years, you probably know that sitting on the couch all day isn't going to make you a healthy person. But what if I told you that even if you adhere to the government's guidelines for daily exercise and work out for thirty to sixty minutes per day three to five days per week, you still may not be doing enough to counteract the damage that sitting for extended periods does to your health? That's a shocking statement for most of us! Don't sit down.

For years doctors, exercise physiologists, personal trainers (like myself), and the government have been telling you that if you eat sensibly, don't smoke or drink to excess and exercise, you could significantly lower your risk of developing heart disease, diabetes, obesity, cancer, metabolic syndrome and a variety of other lifestyle diseases that currently plagues our society. However, new research suggests that although 30 to 60 minutes of exercise per day can help improve lung capacity, strengthen the heart muscle, improve circulation, burn calories, strengthen muscle fibers and connective tissue, lower stress hormones and improve brain function, sitting for long periods of time may be a health risk unto itself, much like smoking tobacco.

The unavoidable truth is that most of us spend the vast majority of our day seated. What I explain in this book is why extended periods of sitting are detrimental to your health, and why you must get up and move regularly, even if only for a minute or two each hour. And what I will show you is how simple it is to fit regular, daily movement into your modern life at work and at home.

I am going to use my wife as an example. My wife is the director of marketing for an architectural millwork company. Her typical day goes something like this: She gets up at about 6:00 a.m. and does twenty minutes of yoga; she showers, gets dressed and gets ready for work. She usually has a couple of cups of coffee and a fruit smoothie for breakfast then drives about seven minutes to work (she is on the low side of commute time, as the average American commute is twenty-three minutes one way to work). She gets into the office at nine o'clock and goes directly to her desk where she proceeds to spend most of the morning working at her computer. About one o'clock she stops and has lunch. Most days she brown bags it, bringing something like tomato soup and a sandwich, or leftovers from dinner the night before, other days she runs out and gets something from a local drive through and takes it back to her desk. The afternoon tends to be more of the same unless she has a meeting. If she has a meeting she might drive to someone else's office and have a seat for that meeting. She usually leaves the office for home at around 6:45. When she gets home she takes the dog for a brisk thirty-minute walk, then we sit down for dinner. After dinner we sit down together on the couch and talk and watch a little television, then toddle off to bed at around eleven.

Does my wife's day sound familiar? It should, because that's pretty typical for most of us. In fact, most of us don't even get in the fifty minutes of exercise my wife fits in. After looking at her typical day, we found that she spent an astounding *twelve hours* in the seated position each day. With this schedule my wife would be considered to have what the government, medical professionals and personal trainers classify as an active life style.

Her fifty minutes of exercise (twenty minutes of yoga and a brisk thirty minutes of walking five days a week) makes her "active," which means she is the poster child for what all of us should be aiming for. But what about all that time that she does nothing but sit? Can those fifty minutes really make up for those other twelve hours? According to several new studies the answer may be no.

The desk job has become the norm in America and across most of the Western world. Many of us are virtually chained to our desks, working on our computers, answering emails, teleconferencing and doing Skype meetings. For most, the only reason to get up out of our chairs is to take a quick bathroom break, and then it's back to the desk to type up that report or send out that follow-up e-mail. According to a poll of 6,300 people by the Institute for Medicine and Public Health, Americans spend an average of 56 hours each week just sitting. That's up by eight percent in the last twenty years. We are also contending with longer commutes to work, leaving us sitting in our car fighting traffic for longer periods of time each day, and causing us to be more sedentary than ever before. But it's not just our jobs that encourage all this sedentary behavior; it's also what we do when we are off work.

Television, or as my father so fondly called it, the "boob tube," has been a favorite after-work pastime since the 1950s. Today, Americans spend 151 hours every month watching television, and most of that time is spent sitting down. Each year the entertainment industry is coming up with more and more reasons for us to have a seat and enjoy an ever-widening variety of entertainment options. My satellite provider boasts more than 250 channels including music, sports and movies along with all the network and cable offerings. That's more than enough to keep the average American glued to the couch almost every night of the week. With websites like Hulu you can stream current and past TV shows at your convenience; add to that video games, social networking sites like Facebook, My Space, Twitter and LinkedIn, and you can see why many of us seem to be growing roots from our butts deep into the couch. What's the big deal you say? So we spend a little more time sitting around. It can't be that bad for us can it? The answer to that question is *yes it can*, and the harm isn't just what it does to your physical health but also the cost to you, your employer and the overall economy.

Inactivity, stress and poor nutrition cause lifestyle diseases that cause more than 300,000 premature deaths, and cost 90 billion dollars in direct health care costs annually, and this doesn't take into account the costs of lowered productivity in the workplace, increased insurance rates and missed workdays caused by illnesses related to inactivity, stress and poor nutrition. But how do we avoid these costs? The official Centers for Disease Control (CDC) guidelines and recommendations for exercise to keep us healthy may not be enough, and most of us have trouble even fitting these minimum recommendations into our busy schedules. On the surface this all sounds like very bad news. I mean, if doing 30 to 60 minutes of exercise isn't enough, then what are you supposed to do? You have to work, but your job has you stuck at your desk. You work hard all day and when you get home you need to unwind and relax. Let's face it, it's enough to make you want to throw up your hands and scream "I quit!" And at times it feels like you may as well just dig a hole and jump in.

Well, I have great news. In this book I am going to give you solutions. Not pie-in-the-sky goals and ideas, but solutions that actually fit into your hectic meeting-filled, gotta-get-that-report-out-yesterday life. I am going to give you real life practical ways to address the physical problem of sitting for too many hours each day. There are movements that you or your employees can really do at their desk in the office, at home or almost anywhere you find yourself seated for more than one hour. The amount of time spent doing these movements will be short; as little as eight minutes in an eight-hour day. Yes, you read that right. Eight minutes. Many of these movements can be done without any special equipment and without spending money. If you're an employer, you can use these techniques to improve your employees' health and lower your health insurance premiums without having to drop a bundle building a gym or yoga studio at you facility. These techniques will also help you or your employees to be more productive, alert and engaged by improving brain function and full body oxygenation. I will also teach you simple stress-reduction techniques that can be done in the office, in a park, or in a restaurant or airport without fear of total and complete public humiliation.

In short, this will be the greatest book you ever read…OK, that's hyperbole. But if you're the CEO or the owner of a business with a group healthcare plan, the simple techniques in this book could save you money on insurance premiums by keeping your employees from getting sick, as well as make your employees more productive and happier by helping them reduce stress. It might even lower the number of sick days your employees take.

If you're a manager, this book will give you ideas that you can take to your boss for employee wellness programs that are cost-effective and simple to implement. Based on cutting-edge research, this won't be one of those rehashed been-there-done-that ideas that everyone at the meeting rolls their eyes at because they've heard it a thousand times. These simple and inexpensive techniques will make you the company hero and maybe, just maybe, get you that raise at your next performance review.

If you're an office worker or work from home, this book will show you how to be healthier, lower your stress levels and improve your focus and productivity. It will also make you feel better and more energetic. It will offer innovative and incredibly simple ways to get more movement into your day without sacrificing any real time. Some of these might seem downright bizarre, but try to keep an open mind. These movements are based in Western science and the emerging field of inactivity studies, as well as the ancient wisdom of Eastern natural health philosophies including Yogic principles and Chinese medicine. And since most of the things you will learn in this book don't require fancy equipment, special workout wear or a lot of space, you probably won't get you a second glance if someone walks by your desk while you're doing them, all of which makes it harder to come up with excuses for why you can't do this.

Now I just want to get this straight from the very start:

THIS IS NOT A WEIGHT-LOSS BOOK. You will not lose twenty-five pounds in twenty-five days by following the advice in this book. Doing one to five minutes of the movements I have created each hour will not give you six-pack abs or a small, tight butt. It will, however, help you be healthier and could quite possibly add years to your life. If you don't currently do any exercise, it can help you get moving and that can start you down the road to a more active, healthy lifestyle. If you already exercise on a regular basis this will get you up and moving more often, which is what research says will counteract the effects of long days and nights of sitting. If you incorporate the information in this book into your life you can *slowly* begin to burn fat with the proper diet. But weight loss is not what this is about.

In fact, this book will barely touch on diet at all. This is not because nutrition isn't important; good nutrition is vital to good health. But there are thousands of great books on diet and nutrition with authors who have far better credentials than I. In fact, check out the appendix of this book for a list of sources that will give you a broad spectrum of thought on nutrition and help you learn to eat healthier for your bio chemistry (yes, I think that diet is *that* complicated). This book was designed to give you (or your employees) what you really want and need to know about how to be a lot healthier, regardless of your current lifestyle.

Chapter 1

In The Beginning

(What the human body was designed to do)

In the beginning there was only darkness, and then there was a big bang. In the blink of an eye, the universe expanded exponentially...OK, that's probably too far back. Let's fast forward a few billion years or so. The time is about 3.6 million years ago and two apelike creatures, one large and one small, are taking a stroll in what is now Tanzania. From the evidence left behind it sounds like it had been a bad week.

For starters, a nearby volcano called Sadiman had erupted earlier and spread a fine layer of ash, similar to beach sand, across the landscape. After the eruption it rained, turning the ash into a wet, almost cement-like substance, perfect for trapping footprints. Enter the apelike creatures. Now these creatures aren't exactly human but they aren't chimpanzees either. These creatures have been dubbed Australopithecus afarensis, and what makes them special is that they walk upright on two feet. We know this because 3.6 million years ago they walked across the African landscape leaving behind 165 of their footprints; footprints that are strikingly different from the prints left behind by chimpanzees, but almost indistinguishable from prints left behind by the likes of you and me. These particular footprints are widely recognized as the first known evidence of primates walking on two feet, or bipedalism. Not long after these early creatures left their tracks in the sand, Sadiman erupted again (no wonder these guys were getting out of Dodge...), laying down another layer of ash and sealing in the footprints for more than three million years. You may be thinking, "ok, that's kind of interesting, but what the heck does it have to do with what my body was designed to do?" In order to answer that question, we have to ask another question. And that question is *"why:"* Why are these Australopiths walking upright in the first place when no other species is?

First off, bipedalism has its advantages. It frees up the arms and hands for tool-making and carrying objects like food, weapons and children for longer distances; It makes us look larger and more imposing; It provides a more efficient walking gait, thus allowing us to cover more territory quickly; and it improves long distance perception. Bipedalism also provides many thermoregulatory advantages which were probably very important on the hot, dry African savanna: A body that is upright has more surface area exposed to wind and rain to help keep it cool and a tall upright posture exposes less surface area to the heat of the sun, especially at midday.

Before bipedalism, our ancestors split their time between the trees and the ground, much like wild apes and chimps do today. While apes and chimps can walk upright for short periods of time, they rely mostly on all four limbs for locomotion. Their bodies were designed to climb trees and they do it very well, but walking around dragging your knuckles is not a very efficient way to get around on the ground. For the same expense of energy, a chimp can knuckle walk six miles while a man can walk upright for eleven. Clearly, if these creatures wanted to venture out of the trees and into new territories, walking on two feet was the way to go.

But why venture out of the trees at all? The apes that stayed in the trees doing what they had been doing for millions of years did fairly well, and some of them are still living that way today. According to Nicholas Wade in his book *Before the Dawn,* there is a legitimate and logical reason:

"So consider this population of 100,000 chimp-like apes somewhere in the eastern side of equatorial Africa 5 million years ago. Times are tough and their forest homeland is shrinking. The trees no longer carry enough fruit. The apes are forced to spend a lot of time on the ground searching for other sources of food. Large cats stalk or ambush the unwary. Each generation is tested by this harsh new environment, and in each generation the better adapted produce more offspring."

He goes on to say,

"There are two kinds of survivor. One, clinging to the remnants of forest, manages to continue in much the same way of life: this is the lineage that leads to chimpanzees, and because it clings to the same habitat it has no great need to change its way of life or physical form. The other manages to survive by venturing into a new niche— it learns to occupy both the trees and the new spaces that have appeared in between them. Helping it survive on the ground is the emergence of a critical new ability — that of walking on two feet."

For a couple million years, give or take, these creatures continued out into the open spaces. They continued to adapt and change as the environment around them changed, taking many different forms, from Homo habilis to Homo erectus, Homo ergaster, Homo genus and Neanderthal. But most importantly, these creatures didn't stand still; they continued to move, exploring Africa and beyond... Well beyond, in fact, into India, Asia, the Middle East and Europe. They did this without horses, donkeys or wheels. The hallmark of early man as a species is that of almost *constant movement*.

About 200,000 years ago, Homo sapiens, or modern man, appeared on the scene. Homo sapiens lived what we now call a hunter-gatherer life style. This lifestyle consisted of looking for wild fruits and plants and hunting or scavenging for animals. This forced them to be constantly on the move; as the season or climate changed they were forced to follow migrations of other animals or search for plants that were ready to bear fruit or were already ripe. As the climate began to change (and change it did, over and over) they were either forced or simply had that same wanderlust that infects many of their modern-day relatives, to move into new territory. From their humble beginnings in eastern Africa these people spread across the globe long before they learned how to farm or domesticate large animals like horses, donkeys or cows. They had not yet invented the wheel so you can imagine that these people were some serious hikers.

While we can't be sure of what happened before written history, we can look at people who lived in a similar way in a similar environment to deduce how our early ancestors might have lived. For example, the hunter-gathers of North America lived very different lifestyles from one coast to the other. Because of their physical environment, east coast tribes like the Powhatan or the Seminole lived quite different lifestyles from the Sioux or the Apache in the west. The eastern tribes as we know from their interaction with the first white settlers in the American colonies were farmers. We've all heard the story of how the pilgrims were saved from starvation by the local Indians who taught them to cultivate corn. The western tribes were mainly hunter-gatherers because the climate dictated that. They hunted buffalo and other game and gathered wild plants. These two different groups living in very different environments did, however, have one significant thing in common: they all had large territories. Some of these territories were as large as hundreds of square miles. Before the reintroduction of horses by European settlers, tribes lived in and travelled throughout these large territories by foot. That, my friends, is a lot of walking.

Early man probably lived in and guarded similar territories when resources became depleted. When another group of people came along and pushed them out, they moved on to new territories. In short, early man's life was full of movement. Their days were spent foraging for food, which included climbing trees for fruit and nuts, digging up roots and tubers, as well as searching for edible plants, insects and honey. Hunting would have been an important part of their daily routine as well. Tracking, killing, cleaning and taking the prize back to the village is physically demanding work. (I can tell you from experience that dragging a dead deer through three miles of dense underbrush back to camp all by yourself will wear you out.) Then there are the daily "housekeeping" tasks, such as gathering firewood, making and fixing tools and hunting gear, keeping the campsite or village clean so as not to attract predators, bringing water back to camp, raising the children and caring for the old. When all is said and done, our ancestors couldn't help but have a very busy and active lifestyle.

Another window into how early man lived was opened in the 1960s by a group of Harvard anthropologists who studied the !Kung tribe of the Kalahari of south central Africa. The archaeological records show that the !Kung's way of life has persisted for thousands of years without a break, making their way of life ancient and intriguing. According to study leader Richard Borshay Lee, as hunter-gatherers, the !Kung diet consisted of 60 to 70% plant-based material they gathered, and 30 to 40% of meat they acquired by hunting (if you're looking for a healthy way to eat, look no further). It took the !Kung between 12 and 22 hours a week to gather all the food they needed to survive. Once you add on the "housekeeping" tasks, their total work week was 40 to 44 hours and almost all of this work was physical in nature.

It is important to note, however, that not all of this work was backbreaking. Sure, splitting logs for firewood or dragging an antelope carcass back to camp was probably really tiring. But tracking the antelope only required you to walk as you followed its tracks or blood trail. Tool-making meant whittling wood into specific shapes and hitting rocks together to make hand axes and arrowheads. But although this work wasn't particularly strenuous, our ancestors did not spend a lot of time sitting around. In fact, sitting around for too long was probably a pretty dangerous activity.

When I was young my grandfather, who was 78 at the time and working full-time at a gas station, was sitting at our dinner table when I asked him why he hadn't retired. He looked at me for a moment, and then shared with me what his grandfather had told him: "If you stand still long enough, Death will find you." He proved himself right when he died within six months of retiring at the age of 81. For early man, the belief that standing still for too long would bring Death a-knocking was undoubtedly true as well. I once took a training course from the U.S. Forestry Service to learn how to be a hike guide, and the first thing we learned was that if you get lost in the forest, then *stay in one place.* Don't wander around trying to find your way out because that makes you difficult to find. If you stay in one place, you are much easier to find. Think about that for a moment: staying in one place makes you much easier to find. In the days of early man, anyone who was looking for you probably wasn't friendly. Whether it was a predator or rival tribe, standing still while they tried to locate you probably wasn't a good idea. Moving frequently served many purposes, one of the most important of which was basic survival.

It was about ten thousand years ago that our nomadic way of life began to change. It was during this time that agriculture was developed. Most experts believe that the agricultural lifestyle started in the fertile crescent of the Middle East where previously wild plants were transplanted, cultivated and harvested for the first time. While this meant that early man spent more time in a single place and less time wandering the landscape, it still kept our ancestors plenty busy. In fact, most scholars agree that during the first Agricultural Revolution, our farmer ancestors spent more time working than did their hunter-gatherer ancestors, and that the work they did was physically more demanding. It is estimated that early farmers spent about 40 hours each week in activity that fed them. Add to that another 40 hours each week spent on activities such as repairing shelters, fences and tools and general maintenance of the homestead. Compared to the !Kung's 40 hours of work per week it seems clear that early farmers were probably even more active than their hunter-gatherer ancestors. Clearing fields, turning soil and planting seeds was backbreaking work. Weeding and keeping birds and insects from destroying crops took lots of time and effort, not to mention harvesting and then preserving or putting those crops into storage. Farming was no easy task. If you are one of those hardy souls who each summer puts in a small garden to help feed your family you know that, even with rototillers and wheelbarrows, maintaining your little ten by ten foot garden plot is physically challenging work.

It was also during this first Agricultural Revolution that man began to domesticate large animals, probably to help with the more physically challenging aspects of farm life, but also for food and clothing. Animals like sheep, goats, pigs, oxen, cattle and horses became very useful. But these animals required care and sustenance and created an additional burden of labor. Our ancestors had to protect their domesticated animals from predators (if you don't believe me ask the ranchers in Montana who even today are squaring off against wolves who attack their sheep and cattle and the environmentalists who want to protect the endangered wolf species) feed them, milk them, shear them and keep them contained so they would not run off. All of these activities kept our ancestor's bodies moving and active, and this way of life would go virtually unchanged for many thousands of years.

But things did eventually change, and drastically so in the mid-1700s as we entered the Industrial Revolution. This change unfolded relatively slowly from a societal standpoint, but in evolutionary terms it occurred in the blink of an eye, which I believe is why we're in trouble today. With each new leap in industrial technology, humans have to do less and less physical labor. This change started simply, especially with agriculture. In the beginning there was a change from wooden tools to more efficient and long-lasting tools made of metal. As the Industrial Revolution progressed into the making of textiles, mining, manufacturing, transportation, steam power and finally back into farming, it would take us from being a principally agricultural society to a manufacturing society. This change would fundamentally alter the way most of us use our bodies, and in a monumental way, would affect our overall health for centuries to come.

Spurred by the Industrial Revolution, scores of people left agrarian lifestyles in the countryside to begin working in factories in the city. As factories began favoring mechanical power over human power, jobs became less about physical activity and more about feeding the machines, moving product from machine to machine, maintaining the machines, and supervising the overall process of manufacturing products. The more advanced the process became, the less active people became until finally the tide turned.

In America, the Industrial Revolution was slow to arrive. With a wealth of land, the country maintained an agricultural society for longer than our European neighbors. But by the early 1900s, the move from wide open spaces to the cities had begun, buoyed by a huge wave of immigrants searching for a better life in the United States. As these people began working in factories and living in cities, their activity levels began to slowly diminish, and as this transition from an active to a largely sedentary lifestyle took place, a new health risk slowly began to rear its ugly head. Before 1900, some of the most feared diseases had been tuberculosis, influenza, cholera, diphtheria and scarlet fever. Cancer, heart disease, stroke, diabetes and obesity were barely blips on the radar screen. But over the last 100 years, these so-called "lifestyle diseases" began to explode. By 1940, lifestyle diseases accounted for more than 60% of all deaths in the United States. These diseases are believed to be caused by the things you eat and drink, environmental influences, tobacco smoke and the amount of physical activity you get; basically things that you have a certain amount of control over. According to numerous studies, the two main culprits in developing lifestyle diseases are diet and physical activity. While both of these are extremely important to a healthy lifestyle, this particular book will focus on the physical activity side of the equation.

During the twentieth century, the importance of physical activity was beginning to be recognized, and a new generation of fitness leaders was born. Men like President Theodore Roosevelt, Jack LaLanne, Kraus and Hirschland, Dr. Thomas K. Cureton and President John F. Kennedy led the charge to popularize, study the effects of, and implement public policy to help improve the health of the American people and bring exercise to the masses. Today the Centers for Disease Control and Prevention (CDC) recommend that you do moderate-intensity aerobic activity for 30 minutes a day, five days a week (or 150 minutes per week). The CDC also recommends two or more days a week of strength training that works all of the major muscle groups. Those are the basics of our current recommended exercise guidelines in the U.S., but the question arises: Is that exercise alone enough?

You may have noticed that until now I have taken great care to use the word "exercise" as little as possible in this book. I have found over the past 25 years as a fitness/wellness professional that the quickest way to get most people's eyes to glaze over and get them looking furtively for the closest exit is to *start talking about exercise*. For many people, the word exercise brings up the same warm, cuddly feelings as words like "root canal" or "IRS audit." But organized exercise or fitness is really a natural progression for a society that is growing more and more sedentary. As our world becomes more mechanized, our daily lives shift to using more and more of our brains and less and less of our brawn. With the advent of modern-day conveniences like escalators, elevators, automobiles, telephones and computers activity is being sucked out of our daily lives (and note, exercise and activity are two different things). We need something to help us keep our bodies moving.

Considering what our bodies were created to do, and the evolutionary history of the human physical experience of regular movement throughout the day, is our "30 minutes five days a week" of exercise all we can do, or even the best thing to do? New evidence says the answer is no. Before you grab your pitchforks and torches to hunt me down and roast me at the stake, allow me to explain. I understand that we are all busy and the thought of adding more to our already heavily-loaded day is not what any of us want. What I'm suggesting is not that we should be doing *more*, but that we should be doing it *differently*, and I will show you how.

Chapter 2

Today

"Things were different when I was coming up." My mother says that a lot and I used to chalk that up to, you know, s**t old people say like "$2.00 for a cup of coffee? Good lord that's a lot of money." Or: "You kids and your cell phones and hula-hoops." But, as much as I hate to admit it, as I began to do research for this book I started to realize just how right my mother is: things really have changed.

In fact, in the last 200 years the way we live our day to day lives has changed more and faster than at any other time in human history. In the year 1812, about 200 years before the publication date of this book, there was no running water in homes, no indoor flushing toilets, no central heating, no electricity in homes or businesses, no trains, planes or automobiles. There were no telephones, radios or televisions. Today all of these things are so commonplace that we barely give them a thought. Progress has definitely marched on and continues to do so. Unfortunately, people aren't doing much marching. All this progress has led us down a path to a very sedentary lifestyle. In fact we spend more time sitting today than at any other time in human history. That includes the young and old, men, women and children. But just how is this affecting our physical health? Take a look at the things we do every day and their impact on our health and our pocketbooks.

Let's begin at the start of our day. After dragging ourselves out of bed and getting ready for work, most of us head off to our car for our daily commute. In the old days this would have been a walk around the forest or savanna looking for food or a short walk from the house to the barn or field when most of us lived a rural life. According to the 2010 U.S. Census Bureau's *American Community Survey*, today's average commute is 25.3 minutes and most Americans now spend more than 100 hours each year commuting back and forth to work. Based on this statistic, we spend more time commuting each year than most of us get in vacation time! In fact, since 1982, the time Americans spend in traffic has jumped an amazing 236 percent.

- The amount of time we spend in our daily commute, which is time spent sitting around, is the perfect example of how modern-day changes are affecting our health. Studies repeatedly show that people making long commutes are at a higher risk for a host of maladies. High blood pressure, sleep deprivation, and depression are at the top of the list. And overall, people with long commutes are fatter, and national increases in commuting time are believed to be one contributor to the obesity epidemic. Researchers at the University of California, Los Angeles, and California State University, Long Beach looked at the relationship between obesity and a number of lifestyle factors, such as physical activity. Vehicle-miles traveled had a stronger correlation with obesity than any other factor.
- In major American cities, the length of the combined morning-evening rush hour has doubled, from under three hours in 1982 to almost six hours today.
- The average driver now spends the equivalent of nearly a full workweek each year stuck in traffic.
- On a typical day, the average married mother with school-age children spends sixty-six minutes making more than five trips and covering twenty-nine miles.
- According to the most recent federal data, the amounts of time mothers spend behind the wheel increased by eleven percent just between 1990 and 1995, and there's every indication that the trend is continuing.
- Moms spend more time driving than they spend dressing, bathing, and feeding a child.
- Stressed-out commuters with little time for loved ones also don't have much time for community involvement.
- Some 42,000 people are killed in auto crashes each year, and three million are injured.

And overall, people with long commutes are fatter, and national increases in commuting time are believed to be one contributor to the obesity epidemic. Researchers at the University of California–Los Angeles, and California State–Long Beach, for instance, looked at the relationship between obesity and a number of lifestyle factors, such as physical activity. Vehicle-miles traveled had a stronger correlation with obesity than any other factor. It's clear that we spend a great deal of time commuting which means a lot of time sitting.

From sitting in our cars during our morning commute, we then make our way into work. We Americans spend a lot of time at work, more time than in any other industrialized nation. According to statistics from the U.S. Department of Labor, workers in the United States clocked in 1,821 hours in 2001, while those in Germany logged 1,467 hours. In addition, the proportion of workers who commuted thirty or more minutes to their jobs increased from 19.6 percent in 1990 to 33.7 percent in 2000. By 2007 that number had increased to 36%. American workers on average spend 45 hours a week at work according to a study by Microsoft Corporation. If you're an executive that number is even higher, where 70-plus hour work weeks are the norm not the exception. That number has been steadily climbing over the past ten years.

To make matters worse, our jobs have become less and less active. According to the Centers for Disease Control and Prevention's weekly *Morbidity and Mortality Report*, most Americans get very little or no physical activity during the work day, and in fact only 6.5% of all U.S. adults meet the "minimum activity guidelines" while at work. To quote my mother, "things were different when I was coming up." A study published in May 2011 by PLos ONE shows that since 1960 jobs that require physical movement have slowly disappeared. Today, less than 20% of private sector jobs require "moderate" activity; that's a whopping 30% less than in the early 1960's. To underscore how sedentary we've become, look at the 2008 study by researchers at the National Institute of Health who had six thousand American adults strap on accelerometers to see just how much they moved over the course of the day (*moved,* not exercised). They determined that less than 5% got in 30 minutes of continuous physical activity five days a week. Equally disturbing is the study published in the *American Journal of Epidemiology* in 2008. This study, which followed 6,329 people, found that 60% of our waking hours are spent in sedentary pursuits like sitting at a desk or driving to work.

What does all of this mean? It means that many of us find ourselves virtually shackled to our desks, hunched over our computers, barely moving for hours on end. The strange thing is, this glued to the chair thing isn't just about being lazy; for many it's about perception. I was reading *Men's Health* magazine the other day and a reader asked the advice columnist if everyone in his office ate their lunch at their computer, should he do the same? The answer surprised me. The advice columnist said that if the reader left the office for lunch, he would probably be seen as the office slacker, even if he's not. I'm guessing that a lot of people are afraid to stray too far from their work space and move around out of fear of being branded a slacker.

Because much of what many of us do for a living today has been consolidated to our computer, wandering away from our chair could immediately be construed as suspicious behavior. I can hear the office talk now:

Ryan: *Where's Josh? He's not at his desk.*

Camille: *He probably just went to the bathroom.*

Ryan: *The bathroom? I saw him in there just a couple of hours ago.*

Janine: *Really? Do you think he has Crohn's disease?*

Camille: *I just said he* might *be in the bathroom. I don't know for sure. I just saw him get up. Maybe he got called into John's office.*

Janine: *The boss' office! Maybe he's getting fired!*

Ryan: *Probably, the guy is never at his desk.*

What I find most interesting about this kind of thinking is that it's not based on any kind of reality. With all the mobile devices available to us today, we can be productive anywhere we happen to find ourselves. Not only that, but if you're a business owner, manager, or a CEO this kind of thinking is costing you big bucks! Study after study shows that the more sedentary your work staff is the more sick days they take, the less productive they are and the higher your insurance costs are. Let me say it again— being sedentary can make you sick! This sitting-at-your-desk-for-hours-on-end thing is not only bad for your health; it is also expensive for you and the company for which you work.

In a perfect world we would all stop at the gym on our way home from work, get in a quick forty-five minutes of cardio, toss around a few weights and do a little stretching. Maybe a couple of days a week we would do a yoga class or shake our groove thing to a Zumba DVD. Then we would get back to the house and whip up a homemade meal with lots of veggies, a little lean protein and some whole grains. Then we would play with the kids and help them with their homework, walk the dog and clean up the house a little. Finally we would head off to bed to get a good solid 8 hours of sleep...and they all lived happily ever after.

Sound like a fairy tale to you? Me too. In the real world, the chances of you stopping at the gym are pretty slim. According to the Bureau of Labor Statistics, only 16% of us will do any kind of exercise on any given day. If you happen to be one of those people that goes to the gym religiously, my hat is off to you. But before you start congratulating yourself and putting this book down to have a protein shake, keep reading into The New

Research chapter, because there is new information you need to know. For the rest of us, we will most likely grab something that is quick and convenient for dinner and then sit down and watch some television, surf the net or spend some time on our favorite social media site. Finally we'll head to bed late and get six or less hours of sleep.

Let's take a look at what the statistics say about how we spend our time at home, starting with television. According to the Nielsen Company, the average American watches more than four hours of TV each day--that's 28 hours per week, or two months of TV-watching per year! In a 65-year lifespan, an average American will have spent nine years glued to the television. *Nine years*...these days, most marriages don't last that long! According to an eye-opening new analysis done by researchers at the University of California, Berkeley, Americans spend nine times as many minutes watching TV or movies as they do participating in sports, exercise and all other leisure-time physical activities combined. When looking at which activities contributed more to energy expenditure among Americans, the researchers found that driving a car, watching TV and working in an office outranked sports and heart-pumping workouts. In this study, which was released by the *International Journal of Behavioral Nutrition,* lead author Linda Dong notes that "[t]his study provides a wake-up call for the nation, particularly in light of rising obesity rates in this country. A lot of people aren't fully aware of how sedentary their lives are. This paper shows that, as a population, leisure-time physical activities are at the bottom of our priority lists." The study provides the first national-scale, quantitative analysis of energy expenditure in the United States. The paper comes during an epidemic of obesity in this country, and at a time when federal health officials are reporting that poor diet and physical inactivity are quickly gaining on smoking as a leading cause of preventable deaths.

So how did the researchers come to find all of this data? The UC Berkeley researchers used data from 7,515 adults questioned from 1992 to 1994 for the National Human Activity Pattern Survey (NHAPS). Those surveyed were asked to report everything they did and how long they did it during the prior twenty-four hours. More than 125,500 reports of activities were grouped into 255 categories that were similar in the energy required to do them. The researchers used information on how many people reported doing each activity, how long they did it, and how much energy it took to do it. From this information, it was possible to estimate total energy expended on each activity. The study found that, outside of sleeping, the largest collective contributor to energy expenditure among the population was driving a car, followed by office work and watching TV, partly because so many people reported those activities. In contrast, leisure-time physical activity, such as jogging or playing basketball, accounted for only 5% of the population's total energy expenditure.

It doesn't take a rocket scientist or a Berkeley researcher for that matter to figure out that cutting back on the time spent watching TV or movies would free up precious minutes for exercise.

But it's not just the television gobbling up our downtime and keeping our butts glued to the couch after we get home from work; social networking sites are fast becoming a popular attraction as well. According to The Nielsen Company, global consumers spent more than five and a half hours on social networking sites like Facebook and Twitter in December 2009, an 82% increase from the same time in December 2008 when users were spending just over three hours on social networking sites. Globally, social networks and blogs are the most popular online category when ranked by average time spent in December, followed by online games and instant messaging. With 206.9 million unique visitors, Facebook was the number one global social networking destination in December 2009, and 67% of global social media users visited the site at least once during the month. The amount of time spent on Facebook has also been on the rise, with global users spending nearly six hours per month on the site. In the U.S., it's not just young Americans using these social networking sites; geezers are now getting seriously into the act as well. According to Nielson, Americans over the age of 50 visited social networking sites twice as often as kids under 18.

So let's see if we can break down all this statistical mumbo jumbo: For the most part it looks like the majority of us spend more time than ever in a seated position trying to get to and from work, and sitting at our desks hunched over a computer screen, only getting up to use the bathroom and eat. Then most of us head home and watch some television or get together with friends via the computer on a social network like Facebook, My Space, LinkedIn or Twitter and we do it all while firmly planted in the seated position. The fact that sitting around isn't very healthy for our bodies really isn't news, but it may surprise you how much this sedentary lifestyle is costing us...above and beyond the price for a new wardrobe because you can't get into your old clothes. The following are the costs for having one of today's most popular lifestyle diseases.

Heart Disease

According to the health website Web MD, in the U.S., all cardiovascular diseases, including heart conditions, stroke, peripheral artery disease, and high blood pressure combined cost $273 billion each year. In fact, of all the money spent in the U.S. on health care, 17% goes toward treating cardiovascular disease, says Paul A. Heidenreich, MD, a cardiologist at the Veterans Administration Palo Alto Health Care System in Palo Alto, California and Associate Professor of Medicine at Stanford University. Heart conditions such as heart failure, heart attack, and surgical procedures such as bypasses account for nearly $96 billion of that total. That, my friends, is a gigantic load of cash.

Ok, so these numbers are figured on a pretty big scale, but what about the costs per person? A recent study published in

Circulation, the *Journal of the American Heart Association* estimated that over the course of one person's lifetime, the cost of severe coronary artery disease -- the most common form of heart disease -- is more than $1 million. That includes both direct and indirect costs. Direct costs, like ambulance transportation, diagnostic tests, hospitalization, and possible surgery and a pacemaker or implantable defibrillator can add up quickly. Long-term maintenance of heart disease is also expensive, including medications, testing, and cardiologist appointments. It's harder to grasp the indirect costs of heart disease, but they can be enormous. The biggest are lost productivity and income. Many people might be able to return to work a few months after having a heart attack, but even losing income for a few months can cause grave financial problems. Surveys show that most people would be only 90 days away from bankruptcy if they stopped getting paid. For people with a severe disease, it can be difficult to return to work full time, and some may never be able to return at all. Even worse, those who don't have good health insurance, or insurance at all, can be financially ruined by heart disease seemingly overnight. Apart from the direct costs, the lost wages alone can be crippling.

Some of you might be thinking to yourself that you don't have to worry about the costs of heart disease; you've had your cholesterol checked and your blood-pressure is in a healthy range. But the truth is, even if you don't develop heart disease, it's still costing you. "You're paying for cardiovascular disease whether you have it or not," Heidenreich says. "You're paying for it in your taxes and your health insurance premiums." He estimates that the average person in the U.S. is paying $878 per year for the societal costs of heart disease.

Diabetes

Diabetes affects nearly 25 million Americans and is the fifth leading cause of death in America, killing more than breast cancer and AIDs combined. According to a report from the Agency for Healthcare Research and Quality, this lifestyle disease is costing Americans $83 billion a year in hospital fees alone, that's 23 % of total hospital spending. According to the 2007 report "Economic Costs of Diabetes in the U.S." the overall cost of diabetes is $174 billion ($116 billion in direct costs like medical expenditures, including drugs, office visits, and hospital costs, and $58 billion in indirect costs such as reduced national productivity). Some other amazing stats:

- One of every five health care dollars is spent caring for someone with diabetes.
- Diabetics have medical expenditures that are 2.3 times higher than other victims of chronic disease.
- Diabetics have more frequent facility stays, more home health visits, and more prescription drug and supply usage.

When you throw in the costs of the hidden diabetes epidemic, that means the 6.3 million people that have the disease but haven't been diagnosed and the 57 million Americans that are considered pre-diabetic (likely to develop type 2 diabetes within 10 years), that $174 billion figure goes up another $43 billion dollars.

According to the authors of the report "The burden of diabetes is imposed on all sectors of society- higher insurance premiums paid by employees and employers, reduced earnings through productivity loss, and reduced overall quality of life for people with diabetes and their families and friends." Interestingly enough, diet and exercise alone can help prevent or control type 2 diabetes, which accounts for 95% of all cases of diabetes, meaning many of these economic and human costs could be saved.

Stroke

While the cost of care for an individual in the first 30 days following a stroke is only $13,019 in mild cases and $20,346 in severe cases, the lifetime cost of a stroke can add up to approximately $140,048. The bulk of those costs come in the form of chronic care and rehabilitation. Although there have been significant decreases in both the mortality rate (20.7% between

1995 and 2005) and the incidence of strokes (12.8% between 1995 and 2006), this trend is expected to soon reverse itself as the population ages – particularly among ethnic minority groups who are at especially high risk of stroke. Providing there are no changes in treatment, preventative care, or trends of risk factors (i.e. incidence of obesity), the result of this reversal will be an increase in spending on stroke care, from $65.6 billion in 2008 to $2.2 trillion by the year 2050.

Cancer

The CDC reports that overall spending on direct care for cancer totaled $74 billion in 2004. While there are no reliable cost projections for cancer, recent years have seen an exponential increase in the cost of cancer drugs, as illustrated in the 2006 *New York Times* article titled "A Cancer Drug's Big Price Rise is Cause for Concern." Cancer treatment is especially prone to spending an exorbitant amount of money on a marginal benefit, with some treatments, such as Avastin – used for metastatic breast, colon, and non-small cell lung cancer – costing over $90,000 for a 1.5-month increase in predicted survival time, or $2,000 per day.

According to the same CDC report, Medicare spent $7.3 billion dollars that year (about ten % of overall cancer spending) on inpatient cancer care, and this total does not even include most chemotherapy, which is administered as an outpatient service and is covered under Part B. Medicare spending on Part B drugs in 2004 totaled $10.87 billion, representing a steady 25% annual increase from the $2.76 billion spent in 1997. Given that the incidence of cancer in people above age 65 is nearly 10 times that of people under 65, as the population ages, Medicare is bound to pay a large and growing portion of the nation's overall spending on cancer treatments. When you consider that chronic diseases account for such a great proportion of Medicare's overall spending, any increases in chronic care spending will directly affect Medicare. This directly affects all Americans because we all contribute to Medicare.

Obesity

The dollar figures for the cost of obesity are high because being obese often leads to having one or more of the other lifestyle diseases. The CDC roughly defines obesity as being 30 pounds over your ideal weight. According to a report published in the online edition of *Health Affairs,* in the United States $147 billion per year is spent on direct medical expenses for obesity, which is just over 9% of all medical spending. Furthermore, obesity is the number two cause of preventable death in the United States. To say that obesity has reached epidemic proportions in the U.S. is actually a bit of an understatement. The numbers are mind-numbing. The Get America Fit Foundation cites the following statistics:

- 58 million Americans are overweight
- 40 million are obese
- 3 million are morbidly obese
- 8 out of 10 over the age of 25 are overweight
- 80% of all type 2 diabetes is related to obesity
- 70% of cardiovascular disease is related to obesity
- Type 2 diabetes costs $63.14 billion per year
- Heart disease costs $6.9 billion per year
- Work days lost due to obesity-related issues cost $39.3 million per year
- Physician office visits cost $62.7 million per year
- Restricted activity days cost $29.9 million per year

The increasing costs of being overweight or obese to individuals, businesses and to society as a whole are astounding. According to a report sponsored by the United Health Foundation and the American Public Health Association, the cost of medical-related expenses from obesity in 2018 could soar to over $344 billion a year. The calculations are based on the projections that, if obesity continues to rise at the current rate, 43% of American adults may be obese. Honestly there are loads more statistics that I could beat you over the head with, but after a while my eyes start to roll back in my head and my teeth hurt.

So let's move on to some happy news. You can save yourself a whole lot of money and even more grief and heartache by doing a few simple things. First, eat a healthy, well-balanced diet, including lots of fruits and vegetables. Personally, I believe in a real food diet that is heavily influenced by the Mediterranean diet, but there are thousands of nutrition books out there so you can find the one that works for you. Next, you need to simply (and I mean SIMPLY) add more frequent and consistent movement to your predominantly sedentary routine over the course of your day to keep these lifestyle diseases at bay.

If you are currently getting 30 to 60 minutes of moderate cardiopulmonary exercise (walking briskly is good enough) 4 to 6 days a week, that's great, but stay with me here, because we're about to go into why it may not be enough. In the next section, we will explore new research that may not only convince you that your chair is definitely causing you harm, but can also help you take the next steps toward making yourself a lot healthier.

Chapter 3

The New Research

Over the years the one thing I have found to be true in life is that things are never as simple as we would like them to be. Just a few years ago if someone asked you if lived an active lifestyle, you knew that if you worked out for 30 to 60 minutes a day 4 to 6 days a week you could answer "yes." If not, you said "I'm working on it." For decades scientists have studied the relationship between how much we exercised and our exercise levels and health. But in the past five years, some scientists began looking at this correlation from a different perspective: Instead of thinking about what *exercise* does *for* the body, researches started to investigate what *sitting* for long periods of time does *to* the body. This was some seriously unconventional thinking.

Rather than looking at what we weren't doing they started to look at what we *were* doing, which was a heck of a lot of sitting. In fact, by some estimates many people are sitting as much as 12 hours a day. This new perspective has begun to turn the science of sedentary studies on its head. Researchers from such diverse fields as epidemiology, molecular biology, biomechanics and physiology are seeing more data that is leading them to believe that the amount of sitting we do on a daily basis may not only be making us very sick, it could be causing us to die prematurely. The most disturbing revelation is that 30-60 minutes of sustained exercise may have little or no positive affect on a sedentary lifestyle. To put it simply, sitting for extended periods of time may be slowly killing you, and just working out after sitting around all day may not be enough to save you.

The fact that sitting around is bad for you isn't very surprising; you would have to be living under a rock not to have heard that doing nothing for long periods of time could make you fat and unhealthy. But most of us thought that if we hopped on a treadmill or took a spin class or shook our groove thing in a Zumba class a few times a week, we'd be cool. But according to microbiologist Marc Hamilton from the University of Missouri we need to adjust our thought process. "People need to understand that the qualitative mechanisms of sitting are completely different from walking or exercising...Sitting too much is not the same as exercising too little. They do completely different things to the body."

In a 2005 article in *Science* magazine, Dr. James A. Levine, an obesity specialist at the Mayo Clinic, gave his insights into why, despite similar diets, some people are fat and others aren't. "We found that people with obesity have a natural predisposition to be attracted to the chair, and that's true even after obese people lose weight," he says. "What fascinates me is that humans evolved over 1.5 million years entirely on the ability to walk and move. And literally 150 years ago, 90% of human endeavor was still agricultural. In a tiny speck of time we've become "chair-sentenced," Levine says. This "chair sentence" as Levine puts it may very well be a death sentence.

So what's the big difference between sitting and standing, you ask? I mean just standing around seems every bit as lazy as sitting, doesn't it? Hamilton knows better. "If you're standing around and puttering, you recruit specialized muscles designed for postural support that never tire," he says. "They're unique in that the nervous system recruits them for low-intensity activity and they're very rich in enzymes." One enzyme, lipoprotein lipase, sucks fat and cholesterol from the blood stream, and burns the fat for energy while shifting the cholesterol from LDL (the bad kind of cholesterol) to HDL (the healthy kind of cholesterol). When you're sitting, the muscles are relaxed, and enzyme activity drops by 90% to 95%, leaving fat to hang out in the bloodstream. After a couple hours of sitting, healthy cholesterol drops by 20%. Amazingly this is just one of the myriad of chemical changes that take place in the body while we sit. Sitting for extended periods of time has a huge cascade of effects on the body, everything from back pain and restricted blood flow to being implicated in an elevated risk of certain kinds of cancer. Let's take a look at what this new research really has to say.

Heart Disease

Heart disease is the number one killer in America today. Most of us feel like if we spend a little time at the gym we can help safeguard our heart from heart disease, but researchers are discovering that the amount of time you exercise and the amount of time you spend on your butt are completely separate factors for heart-disease risk. In fact, new evidence suggests that the more hours a day you sit, the greater your likelihood is of dying an earlier death (regardless of how much you exercise). Believe it or not, it looks like even a sculpted six-pack or a tight tush can't protect you from your chair. In 2009 Dr. Peter Katzmarzyk of the Pennington Biomedical Research Center studied the lifestyles of more than 17,000 men and women, and what he found was both astounding and frightening. The people who sat for most of the day (think computer programmers or customer service reps) were 54% more likely to have a heart event than those who sat almost none of the day (think hotel front desk agents and grocery clerks), and it made no difference how much the sitters weighed or how often they exercised. In Katzmarzyk's words "The evidence that sitting is associated with heart disease is very strong. We see it in people who smoke and people who don't. We see it in people who are regular exercisers and those who aren't. Sitting is an independent risk factor."

So if exercise isn't enough, how exactly do you help protect your heart? A study in the *European Heart Journal* gives us a hint. Genevieve Healy of the University of Queensland in Australia drew on data from 4,757 people who wore tiny accelerometers to measure their movement patterns for seven consecutive days. The information they gathered showed that greater amounts of sedentary time were linked to a wide range of blood markers for heart disease and metabolic disorders. The accelerometers were also able to record breaks as short as a minute that interrupted sedentary time. The number of breaks taken by the subjects throughout the week ranged from 99 to 1,258, and the researchers found that those who took the most breaks were significantly healthier (for example, their waistlines were 4.1 centimetres smaller) than those who took the fewest breaks – independent of the total amount of sedentary time they had accumulated.

The accelerometers recorded not just sedentary time, but breaks in sedentary time as short as one minute long. These breaks were times of movement such as the subject bending over to tie a shoe, fidget, get up to look out the window, or the like. Breaks numbered from 99 to 1,258 per week depending on the subject and their environment. The subjects who moved around the most were significantly healthier than their more sedentary counterparts. In fact, those that moved most frequently had waistlines that were 4.1 centimeters smaller than those who tended to remain sedentary for long stretches of time, regardless of how much total sedentary time each type of subject accumulated.

The general message from this research seems pretty clear: if you want to lower your risk of heart disease, it is vitally important to take frequent, short breaks from your office chair and couch.

To illustrate this point further, in a British study published in 1953, scientists examined two groups of workers: bus drivers and trolley conductors. At first glance, the two occupations appeared to be pretty similar. But while the bus drivers were more likely to be seated for their entire workday, the trolley conductors were running up and down the stairs and aisles of the double-decker trolleys. As it turned out, the bus drivers were nearly twice as likely to die of heart disease as the trolley conductors were. A study published in 2004 that looked at that 1953 study with fresh eyes found that while none of the participants ever exercised, the two groups did sit for different amounts of time. The analysis revealed that even after the scientists accounted for differences in waist size—an indicator of belly fat—the bus drivers were still more likely to die before the conductors did. So the bus drivers were at higher risk of heart disease not simply because their sedentary jobs made them round around the middle, but also because all that sitting truly was making them unhealthy.

Let's revisit the impact of sitting on blood chemistry. In a study reported in the *Journal of the American College of Cardiology*, British researchers monitored 4,512 adults for 4.3 years and found that those who accumulated more than four hours of screen time, basically sitting in front of the TV or computer daily, were twice as likely to be hospitalized or die from a "major cardiac event" compared with those who spent two hours or less. Crucially, this relationship held true no matter how much exercise the subjects got. This data suggests that the problem with too much sitting isn't simply that you don't burn as many calories as you consume. Studies with rats and mice show that any muscle that doesn't contract for several hours starts to undergo harmful metabolic changes.

Over the past decade, scientists have observed that levels of lipoprotein lipase (the enzyme responsible for drawing fat from the bloodstream into muscles, where it is burned as fuel) drop in muscles left idle for too long. When the muscles don't need any fuel, the fat remains in the bloodstream and wreaks havoc elsewhere in the body. This is known as Hyperlipidemia, which means that high levels of fat (or lipids) are in the bloodstream. These fats are important for our bodies to function, but when they are too high, they can put people at risk for heart disease and stroke. Prolonged time spent sitting, independent of physical activity, has been shown to have important metabolic consequences, and may influence triglycerides, high density lipoprotein, cholesterol, fasting plasma glucose, resting blood pressure and leptin, which are biomarkers of obesity and cardiovascular and other chronic diseases.

Travis Saunders, a researcher at the Children's Hospital of Eastern Ontario in Ottawa, Canada, co-authored a recent review paper on this emerging field of study in which he says "[t]he animal research and the few physiological studies that have been done suggest that as long as a muscle is contracting, regardless of how low the intensity is, that seems to prevent you from experiencing some of the metabolic adaptations that happen when you're sedentary." What does all that mean? It means that getting out of your chair and simply walking around or doing simple movements that work on strength, flexibility and balance (like the ones in this book) for short periods of time over the course of the day can keep the fat levels in your bloodstream at healthy levels.

In order to positively affect blood pressure levels, how often and for how long should you stand and do these movements? The jury is still out on this. But according to Joan Vernikos, PhD, former director of NASA's Life Sciences Division and author of the book *Sitting Kills, Moving Heals,*

"Standing up often is what matters, not how long you remain standing. Every time you stand up, the body initiates a shift in fluids, volume, and hormones, and causes muscle contractions to occur; and almost every nerve in the body is stimulated. If you stand up 16 times a day for two minutes, the body would read that as 16 stimuli, whereas if you stood once and remained standing for 32 minutes, it would see that as one stimulus."

Clearly, as relates specifically to blood pressure, frequency of standing is more beneficial than duration.

According to Emmanuel Stamatakis, PhD, MSc, Department of Epidemiology and Public Health, University College London, United Kingdom, "People who spend excessive amounts of time in front of a screen -- primarily watching TV -- are more likely to die of any cause and suffer heart-related problems." He goes on to say, "Our analysis suggests that two or more hours of screen time each day may place someone at greater risk for a cardiac event." This is the first study to examine the association between screen time and cardiovascular events, and to suggest that metabolic factors and inflammation may partly explain the link between prolonged sitting and a risk to heart health.

When compared to those spending less than two hours a day on screen-based entertainment, those who spent four or more hours a day had a 48% increase in risk of all-cause mortality, and those who spent two or more hours a day had an approximately 125% increase in risk of cardiovascular events. These associations were independent of traditional risk factors such as smoking, hypertension, body mass index (BMI), social class and exercise habits. These findings have led many researchers to call for public health guidelines that expressly address what they are calling "recreational sitting" (defined as sitting during non-work hours) in an attempt to counteract the amount of time a large number of working-age adults spend seated while commuting or slouched over a desk or computer for hours at a time while at their jobs. "It is all a matter of habit. Many of us have learned to go back home, turn the TV set on and sit down for several hours -- it's convenient and easy to do. But doing so is bad for the heart and our health in general," said Dr. Stamatakis. "And according to what we know so far, these health risks may not be mitigated by exercise, a finding that underscores the urgent need for public health recommendations to include guidelines for limiting recreational sitting and other sedentary behaviors, in addition to improving physical activity." If you keep up with this sort of thing, you will soon begin to notice that new public health guidelines will talk a great deal more about regular activity. The American Heart Association, the American Diabetes Association, the Canadian government and the Australian government are all considering adding warnings to their guidelines about the health dangers of extended times spent sitting.

Weight Gain & Obesity

If you are struggling with your weight, listen up. The work that Marc Hamilton, PhD and Dr. James Levine are doing points directly to one conclusion: Sitting down is your worst enemy. Even if you look at only healthy people who exercise regularly, the ones who sit the most have larger waistlines and have more unhealthy markers like higher blood pressures, higher blood sugar levels and more heart disease and cancers than those who sit less often. Even more proof that remaining in the seated position for too long adversely affects your waistline even if you exercise. In fact, people who sit for more than three hours each day are just as fat whether they exercise or not. You may be thinking that this is just not possible; after all, the people who are exercising are burning more calories, so it follows that they should be thinner, right? Wrong. Hey baby, the numbers don't lie. The problem is that we burn only a small percentage of calories during exercise. Most of the calorie-burning we do during the day happens not while we are "exercising," but while we are just living our everyday lives. When you spend most of that time sitting, your body's metabolism is basically in hibernation mode. Sitting is one of the most inactive things you can do. You burn more calories standing around twiddling your thumbs or chewing gum than you do just sitting in a chair doing nothing. When you are seated, electrical activity in the muscles drops — "the muscles go as silent as those of a dead horse," Hamilton says, which leads to a series of harmful metabolic effects. Your calorie-burning rate immediately plunges to a third of what it would be if you got up and walked. Insulin effectiveness drops within a single day, and the risk of developing type 2 diabetes rises. So does the risk of being obese. The enzymes responsible for breaking down lipids and triglycerides — for "vacuuming up fat out of the bloodstream," as Hamilton puts it — plunge, which in turn causes the levels of good (HDL) cholesterol to fall.

The average person can burn an extra 60 calories an hour just by standing. Now, you may not be able to stand all day, but if you incorporate one to five minutes of movements every hour that use upper and lower body strength, balance and flexibility in short bursts like the ones in this book, you are right back up there near that 60 calorie mark. These short bursts of movement also keep your body from going into that hibernation mode that happens when you sit without getting up for long periods of time. "But just avoid the chair is the simple recommendation, as much as you can," according to Dr. Hamilton. Ok, so we've got all figured out now, right? The biggest problem with sitting for long periods is that you burn less energy, which makes it easier to gain wait and, conversely, harder to lose weight...or is it? There also seems to be a "physiology of inactivity" that has a cascading effect on lipids, enzymes and body chemistry that is detrimental to our health and may cause us to gain weight. So the problem is two-fold. Not only are we burning fewer calories as we sit but our body is producing-or not producing- chemicals, enzymes and fats that stymie our ability to stay lean and healthy.

This is where many people throw up their hands and say "I'm screwed, just dig a hole and I'll jump in." But there's evidence that the solution to this problem may be a simple one. Another study followed a group of men that normally walked a lot (about 10,000 steps per day, as measured by a pedometer) and were asked to cut back (to about 1350 steps per day) for 2 weeks. By the end of the 2 weeks all of them had become worse at metabolizing sugars and fats. Their distribution of body fat was also changed, meaning they had accumulated more adipose tissue or fat around the middle. In other words, pretty much what you would expect as their activity levels decreased. But another study found that when subjects who sat for extended periods on a regular basis began to take short but frequent breaks to do things, like stand up or stretch and walk around the immediate work space, they had smaller waist lines and better profiles for sugar and fat metabolism than the people who simply sat for long, uninterrupted periods of time. Looking at these two studies together, the people who were walking around regularly and then cut back on their movements got thicker around the middle and saw their blood profiles for sugars and fats become less healthy, while the others improved their waistlines and blood profiles by simply moving around on a regular basis.

These studies all point to the same conclusion: that by simply getting up and moving on a regular basis, you can actually help manage fat gain. The movements I have put together for this book do exactly that and more. By adding resistance training and activating stabilizer muscles for balance, you will be doing more than simply standing and walking around; you will also increase calorie burn and muscle activation. If you combine these short sets of movements for one to five minutes each hour during the work day and in the evening as you watch TV or surf the web with a healthy diet and 30-60 minutes of exercise four to six times a week, you have a great recipe for maintaining your weight and maybe even losing a few pounds. To show just how important these small movements are, Dr. James Levine created the following acronym: "NEAT," short for "non-exercise activity thermogenesis," basically calories people burn doing everyday activities. The reason these activities are so important is that people who seem to do more of them tend to be thinner and people who do fewer tend to be heavier. Even more interesting is that people who tend to be heavier seem to be drawn to do less. According to Dr. Levine's study done at the Mayo Clinic, among people who were obese, "[g]iven an environment that lets people sit for hours and hours a day, they will." During the course of the study, people who were thinner tended to fidget, stand, stretch and walk around more often.

Dr. Levine's study, published in 2005, included 10 men and women considered to be lean, and 10 men and women who were slightly obese. All of them described themselves as being "couch potatoes" and none of them reported exercising much. What the study measured and compared was the subject's non-exercise activity. The researchers then tried to determine whether the subjects' behavior changed when they were put on special diets that were designed to make them gain or lose weight. The subjects wore specially designed underwear equipped with sensors that tracked their posture and every movement at half-second intervals around the clock, yielding as many as 25 million points of data on each participant. To make sure that the researchers got accurate data, dietitians prepared each meal, and every food item was weighed to be sure that every calorie each subject ate was counted.

What researchers discovered was that the lean subjects spent much more time on their feet than the obese subjects. Though it had been previously thought that, because they were heavy, the extra weight made obese subjects less active, the research showed that there was no difference in the activity levels of the obese subjects when they lost weight. They were simply predisposed to being less active. Conversely, the subjects who had been lean and gained weight during the study were no less active, even though they had become heavier. In other words the heavy people did not become more active when they lost weight and the lean people did not become more inactive when they gained weight. Much of this study seems to implicate our habits in determining our activity and fitness levels. The good news is that all habits can be changed. It just takes time and patience.

Nutrition professionals use various equations to calculate the number of calories burned in a day. According to one of these calculations, known as Mifflin-St. Jeor equation, the average man burns about 1750 calories a day and a woman about 1350 calories a day. About 60% of those calories are burned by your body simply staying alive. This is known as your Basal Metabolic Rate or BMR. That is about 1050 calories for a man and 810 calories for a woman. About 30% of our calories are burned in daily activities such as walking around, lifting your arm or tying your shoes-- you know, the basics of your day (not exercise). That comes to 525 calories for men and 405 calories for women. The other 10% are burned eating and digesting food, known as dietary thermogenesis. Now let's look at the average number of calories we burn when we are doing some of the more popular exercise activities (I'm going to try to keep this real by assuming just 30 minutes of exercise because we *all* do that much exercise a day, RIGHT?) Oh, and these calorie burns are based on a 150-pound person. If you weigh more you will burn more calories and if you weigh less you will burn fewer. (These calorie counts for 30 minutes of exercise come to you courtesy of Dummies.com)

Running 10 minute miles 365 cal

Walking 20 minute miles 120 cal

Swimming freestyle 35 yds/min 248 cal

Aerobic dance 342 cal

Bicycling at 12 mph 283 cal

Golf (carrying your bag) 174 cal

You will notice that most of us will have burned more calories just doing the everyday things than you did during the 30 minutes of exercise. Now that doesn't mean you shouldn't do the exercise, but what if you did the exercise and increased the amount of movement you did during the regular part of your day?

Diabetes

According to the American Diabetes Association "diabetes mellitus or simply, diabetes is a group of diseases characterized by high blood glucose levels that result from defects in the body's ability to produce and/or use insulin." You may have noticed the phrase "group of diseases." There are two types of diabetes, type 1 and type 2. Type 1 is usually diagnosed in children and young adults. In type 1 diabetes the body, due to some genetic flaw or damage caused by another disease, does not produce insulin. Insulin is a hormone that is necessary to convert sugar, starches and other nutrients into energy. To make this a little easier to understand, let's break it down. When you chow down lunch, your body breaks down that number 3 combo from your favorite burger joint into components that it can use to fuel and repair the body. The starches and sugars are broken down into glucose which the body uses as energy. Insulin takes the sugars from the blood into the cells themselves. But when the body doesn't produce enough insulin or the cells ignore it, the glucose builds up in the blood, which can lead to diabetic complications. Only about 5% of people with diabetes have this form of the disease. Type 2 diabetes on the other hand, is considered "lifestyle-related," and is the most common form of the disease. With type 2 diabetes, either the body doesn't produce enough insulin or the cells simply ignore the insulin. Literally millions of Americans have been diagnosed with type 2 diabetes and those numbers are growing every day. Amazingly, an even greater number of people are at risk of developing type 2 diabetes and don't even know it.

So what in the world does sitting for long periods of time have to do with diabetes? Our health is so incredibly interconnected; one thing just seems to lead to another. The more you sit the fewer muscles you use. The fewer muscles you use, the less energy you burn. The less energy you burn, the more of the calories that you ingest are stored as fat. The more fat is stored up in the system, the more glucose ends up in the blood stream, which can lead to type 2 diabetes. All of the things we talked about in the heart disease and weight gain/obesity sections apply here as well, so make sure that you read those two sections thoroughly. But with diabetes your daily activity is even more important, because how and when you burn your calories makes a real difference. Remember what Dr. Hamilton said about exercising and a sedentary life style? This is especially true for diabetics. A sedentary lifestyle is precisely what contributes most to a person's risk of developing diabetes and that person's subsequent ability to manage the disease after they have been diagnosed. You can run two or three miles a day and lift weights until you have to be carried out of the gym, but if your posterior is firmly planted in that office chair for the majority of the day, you may still be at risk for type 2 diabetes or have trouble controlling the disease if you already have it.

With very little effort you could increase the number of calories you burn and do a better job of regulating the amount of fats and most importantly for diabetics and pre-diabetics, blood glucose levels throughout the day.

Cancer

According to the American Institute for Cancer Research, nearly 100,000 cases of cancer could be prevented if we just spent less time sitting around. Dr. Neville Owen, PhD says "sitting is emerging as a strong candidate for being a cancer risk factor in its own right...It seems highly likely that the longer you sit, the higher your risk. The phenomenon isn't dependent on body weight or how much you exercise." Researchers estimated that as many as 49,000 cases of breast cancer and 43,000 cases of colon cancer each year can be linked to a lack of physical activity. To explore the association between sitting time and mortality, researchers led by Alpa Patel, Ph.D. analyzed survey responses from 123,216 individuals (53,440 men and 69,776 women) who had no history of cancer, heart attack, stroke, or emphysema/other lung disease enrolled in the American Cancer Society's Cancer Prevention II study in 1992. They examined the amount of time spent sitting and physical activity in relation to mortality between 1993 and 2006. They found that more leisure time spent sitting was associated with higher risk of mortality, particularly in women. Women who reported more than six hours per day of sitting were 37% more likely to die during the time period studied than those who sat fewer than three hours a day. Men who sat more than six hours a day were 18% more likely to die than those who sat fewer than three hours per day. Women and men who both sat more and were less physical were 94% and 48% more likely, respectively, to die during the time period studied compared with those who reported sitting the least and being most active. Associations were stronger for cardiovascular disease mortality than for cancer mortality.

Back Pain

Back pain is not a life-threatening disease, but having chronic back pain can make life pretty unbearable. Take it from a guy who broke his back at the tender age of 19, was a paraplegic for a year, and has dealt with back pain ever since. The chair you're sitting in right now probably isn't helping you much if you suffer from back pain, even if it is super expensive and says it's ergonomically correct.

"Short of sitting on a spike, you can't do much worse than a standard office chair," says Dr. Galen Cranz, a professor of environmental design at the University of California at Berkeley. The problem is that the spine simply wasn't designed to stay in the seated position for long periods of time. For the most part, the slight S shape of the spine serves us well. "If you think about a heavy weight on a C or S, which is going to collapse more easily?

The C," she says. But when you sit, the lower portion of the back known as the lumbar spine has its curve collapse, turning the spine's natural S-shape into a C, hampering the core musculature that support the body. The body ends up slouching and the muscles through the ribcage and all of the postural muscles lose their strength and cease to function properly from lack of use, leaving you out of balance and in a poor spinal position, and *voilà*: back pain.

This, in turn, causes problems with other parts of the body. "When you're standing, you're bearing weight through the hips, knees, and ankles," says Dr. Andrew C. Hecht, co-chief of spinal surgery at Mount Sinai Medical Center. "When you're sitting, you're bearing all that weight through the pelvis and spine, and it puts the highest pressure on your back discs. Looking at MRIs, even sitting with perfect posture causes serious pressure on your back."

My good friend Dr. Logan Osland, a chiropractor in Ventura, California sees patients every day that are in severe pain because of sitting for most of their day. "As a chiropractor I talk to people on a daily basis about how bad it is to sit all the time," Dr. Osland says. "From just a mechanical perspective, our core and gluteal musculature activity volume decreases dramatically. Our anterior hip musculature becomes tight from being in a constant shortened position. As a result our low backs have to take on more responsibility for movement, which eventually causes injury." But us isn't just our lower back that is affected by long bouts of sitting. According to Dr. Osland, sitting can also have negative repercussions on the neck, shoulders, and mid-back. "The problem for these areas is everything is out in front of us. Our back is stabilized, causing vertebrae to become immobile; the shoulder blades move out wider; arms internally rotate; neck becomes straight and the head moves forward." In chiropractic terms this is referred to as FHP, or forward head posture. FHP can lead to headaches, neck pain, and upper-extremity nerve entrapment syndromes (like carpal tunnel and cubital tunnel). According to Dr. Osland, "low back pain is the second leading cause of missed work days, second only to the common cold."

What's obvious here is that sitting is not good for spinal alignment, and since the spine houses the spinal cord which sends all the messages from the brain to the rest of the body, spinal alignment is pretty darned important. The only way to relieve the pressures on the spine caused by sitting is to get up and move. This forces the postural muscles to activate, allows blood to flow through the spinal region, and gets us back to moving the way that nature intended.

Another colleague, Breena Maggio, Restorative Exercise Specialist and owner of "The Body Education Alignment Center for Health" in Ventura, California puts it this way:"Many people don't realize that the detriment of sitting is not just in the not moving, but in these two primary things: 1) the change to the resting length of the muscles that happens when the body is in a static position for 8-16 hours per day, every day and 2) the change to the geometry of your blood vessels from maintaining this static position for hours on end, which affects how your blood flows through your blood vessels. Most people also don't realize just how many hours per day then spend in a sitting position of hip and knee flexion (think work, driving, exercise machines, bikes, couches, mealtimes)- count them, you'll be surprised. "

My wife certainly was. As I mention in the introduction, we tracked her time spent sitting and were flabbergasted at the total. Maggio goes on to say,

"First, to address the change in resting length of the muscles: Your body (every single system, tissue and cell) works best, when it is aligned as nature intended. We are designed to be moving creatures, not static creatures, and movement is different from exercise. To maintain this optimal alignment requires all of your muscles. That's ALL of them, not just the 12 or so major muscles you work at the gym, to be at their correct length."

This means that the little postural and stabilizer muscles are just as important as the big muscles.

"When your body is in one position for many hours per day, this is your training program. Your hamstrings, calves, and hip flexors are in a chronically shortened position and you are training them to maintain this shortened position. The flip side of this is that to be able to stand up in alignment and walk optimally, you need your hamstrings, calves, and hip flexors to be at their optimal length."

She continues,

"Muscles that are too short are muscles that have very little innervation. And muscles that are lowly innervated use less energy and have less space to carry blood, which means higher blood pressure overall in your cardiovascular system. It also means, if you have great quantities of muscle that you are not able to use because the muscles are not innervated, you have a lower basal metabolic rate (metabolism) than you should have. Metabolic Syndrome anyone? Diabetes? Obesity? It really is amazing, but it's true: Stretching alone (proper stretching) can be the best weight loss program you've ever tried."

"Second, the change in the geometry of your blood vessels is a bigger contributor- actually it's the major contributor- to the increased risk of death. The reason that sitting increases the risk of death is much simpler than the fat, cholesterol, and chemistry that we are trying to make it...it's about geometry. Your body's circulatory system is arranged in such a way to maximize optimal blood flow. When you add random twists and turns to your blood vessels, which you do with chronic sitting, you affect the flow of your blood. What actually is happening on the cellular level, is an increase in the number and frequency of "wall wounding". This is what causes plaques to form on the arterial walls. A blood cell bangs up against the blood vessel wall and creates a wound. This is the first stage of plaque accumulation. Allow this to keep happening over and over again, and you've got yourself some cardiovascular disease. Exercise doesn't affect the wall wound or the wounding itself. But you can change your blood vessel geometry for the good and stop the wounding just as easily as you bent it all up when you sat down."

"Stand up. When you stand up, you remove all the arbitrary bends and curves you created when you sat down. Understand that if you've been sitting for many hours, for many days, for many years, your muscles, and thus your bones and joints, are not yet ready to jump up and stand for 8 hours straight. You need to add the necessary stretching. Start with a simple calf stretch done using a half foam roller. Do this multiple times throughout the day. Heck, you're already standing, it's easy to stretch your calves at the same time. Actually, the best thing you can do for your body is to change positions frequently. You can sit when you need to. Stand for part of the time. Even squat. Yes, I said squat. Can you sit on the floor for part of your workday?"

"Unfortunately, despite what fitness and the media have been telling us for years, we cannot make up for not moving and undo the chronic sitting position we hold our bodies in for 8-16 hours per day, with a short bout of intense exercise. It's impossible. This is why, in the studies done on the deadly effects of sitting, those who exercised and those who did not, were at equal increased risk of death. Exercise does not undo the damage done by the change to the muscles length and the blood vessel geometry. Therefore, sitting on an exercise bike to do your work isn't going to undo it either. Also, since the only way to walk on a treadmill is to flex at the hip and put one leg out in front, this is not the solution to undoing all that sitting hip flexion either."

Maggio concludes,

"Some of the changes you'll need to make are contrary to what you think you can do. But you're going to have to think a little differently about what is "normal" or what your coworkers will think if you want to save yourself from your maniacal killer chair."

Although this research is very much in its infancy, scientists and researchers all over the world are delving into the effects of sitting for extended periods of time on the human body and our overall health. As more of this research comes in, we will get a clearer picture of exactly how much we need to move to stay healthy and lower our risk of developing ailments like heart disease, diabetes, obesity and cancer. But what is clear even today is that our bodies were designed to be, and need to be, active on a regular basis, and for many of us our current lifestyle is not keeping up with those very basic needs. If you're a "the glass is half empty" kind of person, you might be thinking that this is just more bad news—just another group of scientists with the voice of doom and gloom predicting our early demise. But that's not the case at all. Our technology has lead us down a road that turned out to be a bit of a dead end health-wise, but we haven't traveled very far down that road, and getting back on the right track won't take much time. The real message here is that the fix is an incredibly easy one. This simple fix will make you feel better and more energized. It will make you more productive, lengthen your life and lessen your pain, and you can accomplish all that by just standing up! And if you can do all that by just standing up, think of what you could accomplish if you did movements that improved your strength, balance, flexibility and energy. We aren't talking about hours of drudgery here. We're talking just minutes a day! I'm not sure how the news could get any better, unless of course it came in a pill--but nothing worth having is that easy. So now it is time to stand up for your health, literally! In the next chapter you will learn simple movements that can help you in many ways, but you have to be willing to take the first step. What are you waiting for? Let's get started!

Chapter 4

Introduction to Movement

In the next section of this book you will find descriptions and photos of movements I have created that can be done at home, in your office, cubicle or at your desk. You won't need any special equipment or clothing (although some of the movements may be challenging in tight skirts, and if you wear high heels I suggest you remove them before doing the movements. That goes for you guys, too). These movements were created to be office-friendly, so you won't have to get down on the floor to perform these movements, and you shouldn't get too many stares from your co-workers or be dripping with sweat when you're done.

The movements were designed not only to help you get your body up and moving but also to improve flexibility, balance and strength, and energize your body and mind. Try not to worry that you're taking time away from your assignments; these short movement breaks have been proven to make you more alert and productive over the course of your day, so you'll actually make more progress and be more effective when you get back to it. To make this as user-friendly as possible, I have listed the movements individually under categories of benefits, such as *strength* or *balance*, kind of like the à la carte menu at your favorite bistro. So if you want, you can chose the individual movements that meet your needs at any given time and put them together as you see fit.

Following the menu of movements, you will find a section of "activity segments," which are groups of individual movements that will take one minute, three minutes or five minutes. So let's say you're just beginning and you want to start out on the lower end of the curve. Go to the "One Minute" segments and choose a group of movements. I'll tell you what movement to do and exactly how long to do each movement, which will help those of you who want or need a little more structure. Along with the basic benefits, each of these activity segments has been given a name so it can be easily identified. All you have to do is just follow the directions and after one minute, you'll be back at your desk feeling perky again. Next hour, you might find that you can spare three minutes, so you would just choose one of the "Three Minute" segments and, well, you get the picture.

> *Here's a tip: To get into the habit of getting your butt out of the chair every hour, you might want to set the alarm on your cell phone (on vibrate so as not to be disruptive to your co-workers) and keep this book open to the activity segment you plan to do next. And don't spend a bunch of time preparing—just get moving!*

I spent hundreds of hours choosing movements from traditional fitness, yoga, Pilates, Tai chi and Qi gong. I've even created a few new ones myself, all of which made me feel very important... almost guru-like. (My wife loves when I use *that* line). But the truth is, even if all you do is get up every hour and head to the water cooler, stand up and do a few stretches, or head up the stairs to chat with the IT department about the speed of your computer, you are going to be way ahead in your quest to be healthier.

By doing these simple movements on a regular basis you can help develop your body's many capabilities such as strength, flexibility and balance, and these are just a part of what you need to do to improve your health. Regular extended exercise (30 to 60 minutes four to six times per week) is critical to your long-term health. Cardiopulmonary exercise (like walking, jogging, swimming, or biking) and strength training (weights, bands, push-ups, rock climbing, etc.) improves blood flow and bone density, strengthens the heart and lungs, helps control weight, improves mood, boosts energy levels and improves cognitive function, among other positive health benefits for the body.

If you don't currently do 30 to 60 minutes of exercise four to six days a week, then you should start, and doing these simple movements for one to five minutes every hour is a great way to begin down that road. If you currently do work out on a regular basis, congratulations! Adding these movements to what you are already doing will help you combat the toll taken on your body by extended amounts of sitting.

And now for the fine print: **Before starting this or any other fitness program you should talk to your health care provider to be sure the movements are safe for you.** (My lawyer made me say that).

Well, what are you waiting for? Let's get started!

Chapter 5

Menu of Movements

As you go through the movement section of this book and try out the movements, keep in mind that breathing is very important. Of course it is—try holding your breath for a full minute—which is exactly my point: Don't hold your breath. It is important to keep breathing throughout the entire time that you are doing these movements.

Flexibility Movements

Chair-Supported Downward Facing Dog

Rise from your seated position and walk behind your chair. Secure the chair so that it will not move or roll away. Facing the back of the chair, grab the top of the chair back and then take a step or two backwards away from the chair until your arms are fully extended. Hinge at the hips and lean forward, bringing the torso parallel to the floor beneath you. You should feel a gentle stretch in the low back and hamstring muscles. Hold for 30 seconds.

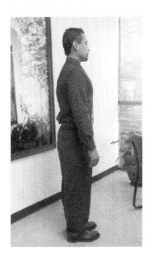
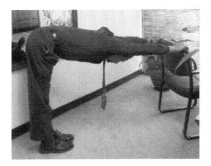

Modified Hanging Pose

Begin in a standing position with feet hip distance apart. Bend both knees slightly, then lean forward and slowly lower your head as you begin to reach down toward your mid-thighs or knees depending on what feels comfortable for you. Support the upper body with your hands, and allow the spine to lengthen toward the floor as much as feels comfortable. Hold this pose for 5 long, slow, deep breaths.

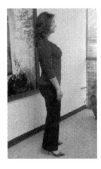 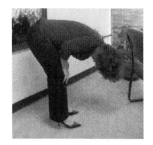

Turning the Head

Begin in a standing position with arms hanging at your sides and the palms of your hands facing your body. *Very slowly* turn your head to the right and look over your right shoulder as you rotate the palms of your hands out so that they point out and away from your body. *Very slowly* turn your head back so that you are looking forward again as you rotate your palms back so that they face your body again. *Very slowly* turn your head to the left and look over your left shoulder as you rotate your palms out so that they point out and away from your body. *Very slowly* turn your head back so that you are looking forward again as you rotate your palms back so that they face your body again.

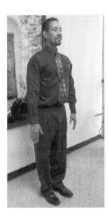 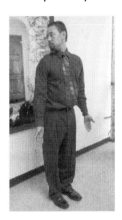

Baby Camel Prays to the Gods

From a standing position place your hands on the front of your thighs for support, then lean forward as you roll your shoulders inward and round the back, dropping your chin down to your chest creating a humped back. Pause for a moment, and then one vertebra at a time bring yourself back up to your standing position bringing your arms down to your sides. Slowly roll your shoulders back, lift the chest and look to the sky.

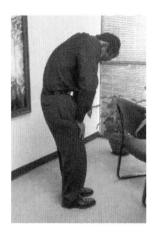
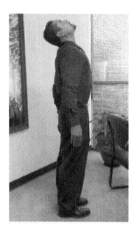

Hip Swivels

Stand with your feet hip distance apart. Place your hands on your hips and slowly start to roll your hips in a circle. With each swivel of your hips make the circles a little bigger. After 10 seconds, switch directions.

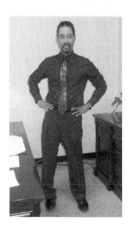
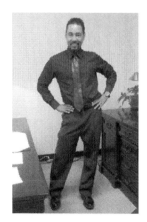

Shoulder Rolls

Stand with your feet hip distance apart, arms hanging down to your sides. Gently roll the shoulders forward, down and back making as big a circle with the shoulders as you comfortably can. After 5 or 10 seconds, reverse the direction of your circles.

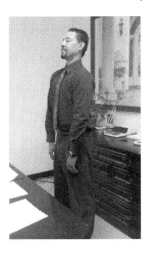 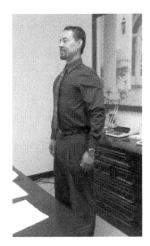

Neck Rolls

Stand with your feet hip distance apart, arms hanging down to your sides. Gently roll your head in small circles and then slowly make each circle a little bigger. After 5 or 10 seconds, reverse the direction of your circles.

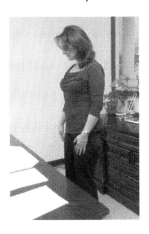 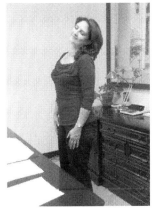

Pec (pectoral) Stretch

From a standing position bring both hands together behind your back and interlace the fingers. Press your chest out as you lift the joined hands upward, towards the backs of your shoulders. Hold for 10 seconds.

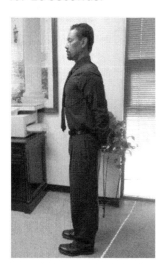 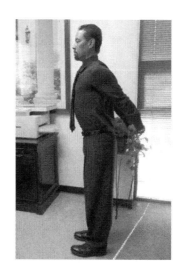

Quad & Hip Flexor Stretch

Stand and hold onto a chair or your desk with your left hand. Bend your right knee bringing your right heel up towards your buttocks. Reach down and grab your right ankle. Pull your knee cap down towards the floor and press your right hip gently forward. Hold for 5 to 10 seconds. Switch sides.

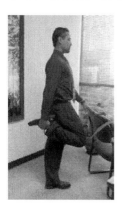 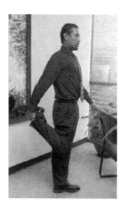

Calf Stretch

From a standing position turn and face your desk or wall. Place the palms of your hands on the desk or wall and bend your left knee slightly as you take your right foot and step back. Press your heel down towards the ground and lean gently forward. You should feel a gentle stretch at the back of your lower right leg. Hold for 5 to 10 seconds then switch legs.

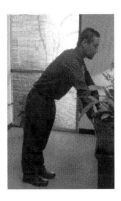 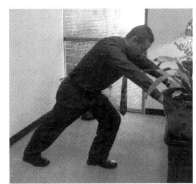

Half Eagle

You can do this one from either the standing or seated position. Bring your left arm directly out in front of you at chest level, bend the elbow and point your forearm and hand up towards the sky. Take your right arm and cross the right bicep under your left elbow as you reach with your right hand up and around your left forearm grabbing the inside of the left wrist. Hold for 5 to 10 seconds then switch sides.

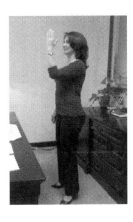 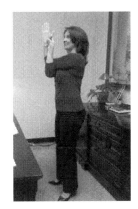

Triceps Stretch

You can do this one from either the standing or seated position. Reach up towards the ceiling with your right arm then drop your right hand down behind your head, pointing your right elbow up towards the ceiling. Reach up to your right elbow with your left hand and gently pull the elbow towards the midline of your body until you feel a gentle stretch in the back of your right tricep. Hold for 5 to 10 seconds then switch arms.

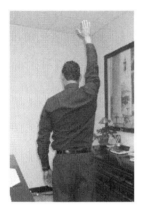 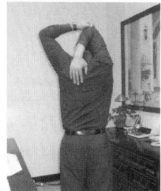

Hamstring Stretch

From a standing position step forward with your right foot approximately 2 feet keeping your right knee straight but not locked. Hinge at the hips, leaning forward until you feel a gentle stretch in the back of the right thigh. Hold for 5 to 10 seconds and switch legs.

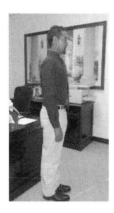 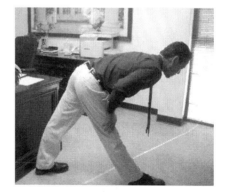

Side-Step Lunge

Begin in a standing position with feet hip distance apart. Step with the right foot to the right about 12 inches. Keep the left knee straight and bend the right knee, leaning out towards your right foot until you feel a gentle stretch on the inside of your left leg. Hold for 5 to 10 seconds then switch sides.

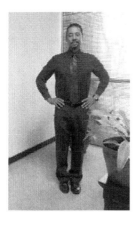 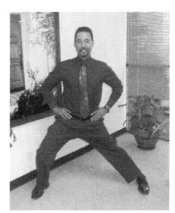

The Archway

Begin by standing in front of a stable desk or chair. Turn your back to the desk or chair and place the palms of your hands on the desk or chair behind you with your fingers pointed away from your body. Keeping your hands on the desk or chair, take a short step away with both feet, then arch your back and press your chest up towards the ceiling. Gently drop your head back and look up at the ceiling. Hold for 10 seconds and then walk your feet back to the original position.

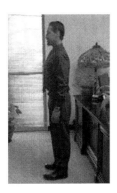 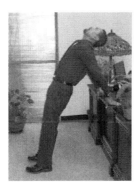

Round and Open *(you don't even have to get up for this one!)*

Sitting in a chair with your feet on the floor, begin by bringing your shoulders directly above your hips, lengthening your spine upward as your head floats away from your shoulders. Drop your chin down to your chest and slowly lean forward as you roll the shoulders in towards the chest, making an exaggerated hump in your back. Bring your forearms to the fronts of your thighs as you pull the shoulder blades apart. Hold for 30 seconds as you breathe.

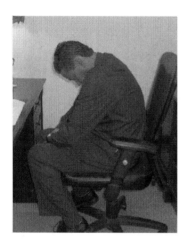 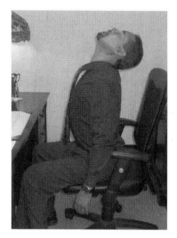

Now, slowly, one vertebra at a time, bring yourself back up to a tall seated position, then roll your shoulders back, open the chest, arch the back and look up to the ceiling. Breathe deeply as you let your arms drop down to your sides.. Hold for 30 seconds and come back to the tall seated position.

Seated Forward Fold *(you don't have to get up for this one either!)*

Begin in a tall seated position with your feet about hip distance apart Hinge at the hips as you lean forward from the waist. Drape the front of your torso over the front of your thighs, dropping your head between your knees, and grab hold of your ankles. Let your head drop and dangle, relaxing your neck. Pull your lower spine away from your hips. You should feel a gentle stretch in your lower- and mid-back. Hold for 30 seconds and return to your tall seated position.

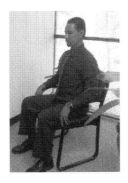 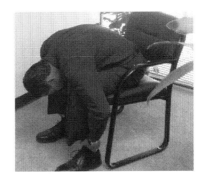

Sitting Man-Style

Begin in a tall seated position. Cross your right ankle over your left knee, creating a triangle shape with your right leg, then gently press down on the inside of your right knee until you feel a gentle stretch through the hip and buttocks. Hold for 30 seconds. Now gently lean forward, bringing the chest down towards the legs; this should intensify the stretch. Hold for another 30 seconds. Switch sides and repeat on the other side, then return to your tall seated position.

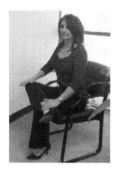 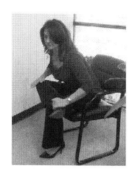

Seated Twist

Begin in a tall seated position. With both feet on the floor, gently turn to the right keeping your spine long, yet relaxed. With your right arm, reach to the back of your chair as you twist the torso using the back of the chair as leverage. Without straining your neck, turn your head and torso as if you were going to look behind you. Hold for 30 seconds. Repeat on the opposite side. Return to your tall seated position.

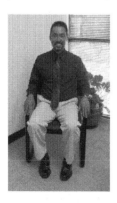 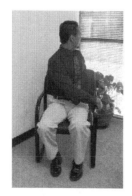

Cross Legged Seated Twist

Begin in a tall seated position. Cross your right leg tightly over the left as if you were wearing a short skirt or kilt. Gently turn to the right, keeping your spine long yet relaxed. With your right arm, reach to the back of your chair as you twist the torso, using the back of the chair as leverage. With your left hand gently press your knees towards the left side of the chair. Without straining the neck, turn your head and torso as if you were going to look behind you. Hold for 30 seconds. Repeat on the opposite side. Return to the tall seated position.

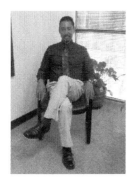 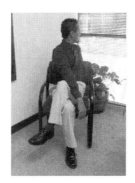

Balance Movements

All of these movements can be done while steadying yourself on an immovable object.

Wu Chi Stance

Stand with your feet slightly wider than hip distance apart. Bend your knees slightly (the deeper you bend your knees the more challenging this exercise becomes). Now tuck your tailbone under the spine, lengthening the lower back. Let your arms dangle at your sides. Roll your shoulders gently open and relax the chest. Allow your head to float off your shoulders. Hold for 30 seconds.

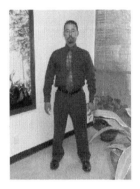 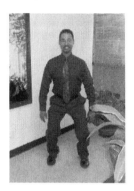

Dog Wags His Tail (Modified)

From Wu Chi Stance, bring your hands down to the fronts of your thighs and rest them there. Bend your knees a little deeper, but be sure to keep the tailbone tucked under the spine, lower back long. Now slowly shift all of your weight over to your right foot and pause there for a moment (for more of a challenge, lift your left heel off the ground with only the toe touching).Then with both feet firmly on the ground again shift your weight over to your left foot and pause for a moment (you can lift the right heel if you wish). Go back and forth between the two feet 3 or 4 times.

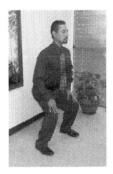 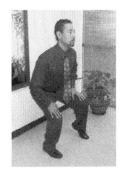

Sumo Step

Stand with legs twice hip width apart. Drop the buttocks down six to 10 inches bringing you into a wide legged squat position (the deeper the squat the more challenging this becomes). Shift your weight over to your right foot and slowly lift your left foot off the ground 1 to 8 inches. Hold for a count of 5 then slowly lower the left foot back to the ground. Repeat on the opposite side.

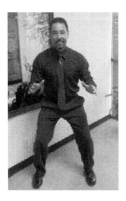 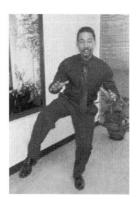

Ankle Circles

Stand with your feet hip distance apart. Shift all of your weight onto your left foot and slowly lift your right foot off the ground. Balance there on your left foot for a breath or two then slowly roll the right foot in a circle for 5 seconds. Slowly bring the right foot back down to the ground and repeat with the left foot.

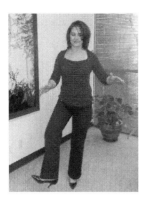 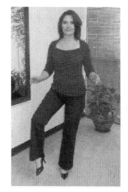

Lifting the Knee

Stand with your feet hip distance apart. Shift all your weight onto your left foot and slowly lift your right foot off the ground. Bring your knee up slowly until it is even with your hip (thigh should be parallel to the floor), then slowly lower it back down to the floor. Switch legs.

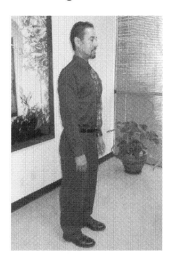 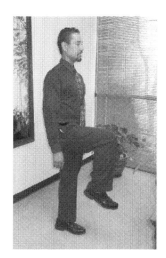

Empty Step

Stand with your feet hip distance apart. Shift all of your weight onto your left foot and slowly lift your right foot off the ground. Bring your knee up slowly until it is even with your hip. Extend your right foot and bend your left knee, touching the toe of your right foot on the floor about 12 inches in front of you, putting no weight on the right foot (as if you were testing the temperature of the water in a lake you were thinking of swimming in). Lift the knee back up to hip level then return to your starting position. Switch legs.

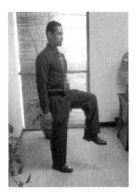 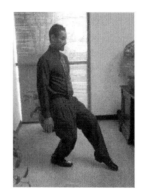

Raising your Internal Temperature

Stand with your feet hip distance apart. Begin to march in place very slowly, raising your right leg to a slow count of 3 then lowering it to a slow count of 3, then do the same with the left foot. Continue alternating for 10 to 20 seconds.

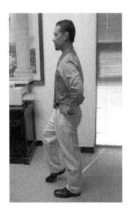 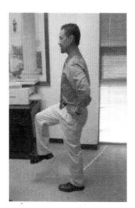

Tree Pose (modified)

Stand with your feet hip distance apart. Shift your weight onto your left foot and bring your right foot off the ground. Place the sole of your right foot against the calf of your left leg. Bring the palms of your hands together in prayer position in the middle of your chest then forcefully push them together. Hold for 10 seconds then switch legs.

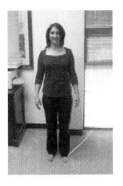 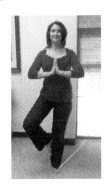

Standing Single Leg Circles

Stand with your feet hip distance apart, with your desk or a chair that will not move directly to your left. Place your left hand on your desk or chair to steady yourself, then shift all your weight onto your left foot, keeping your torso erect and spine tall. Lift your right leg out to the side pointing your toe at the floor (your foot should be about 6 inches off the floor). Make a circle with your foot about the size of a volleyball for 10 seconds. Switch sides.

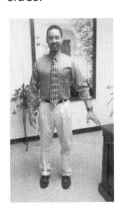 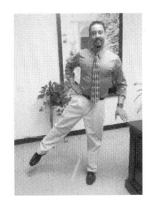

Standing Single Leg Back Beats

Stand with your feet hip distance apart with your desk or a chair that will not move directly to your left. Place your left hand on your desk or chair to steady yourself then shift all your weight onto your left foot, keeping your torso erect and spine tall. Lift your right leg backwards as you point the toe. Lift your foot anywhere from 1 to 12 inches off the floor (the higher you lift the leg the more difficult the movement). Drop your foot down to the floor and lightly touch the toe on the ground then lift it again. Repeat for 10 seconds then switch sides.

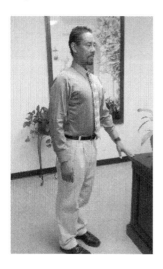 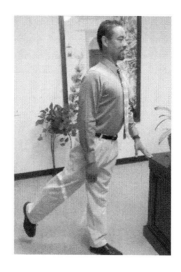

Standing Single Leg Side Beats

Stand with your feet hip distance apart with your desk or a chair that will not move directly to your left. Place your left hand on your desk or chair to steady yourself then shift all your weight onto your left foot, keeping your torso erect and spine tall. Lift your right leg sideways (out to the right of your body) as you point the toe. Lift your foot anywhere from 1 to 12 inches off the floor (the higher you lift the leg the more difficult the movement). Drop your foot down to the floor and lightly touch the toe on the ground then lift it again. Repeat for 10 seconds then switch sides.

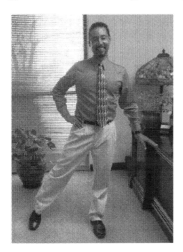 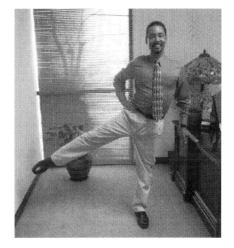

Standing Single Leg Front Beats

Stand with your feet hip distance apart with your desk or a chair that will not move directly to your left. Place your left hand on your desk or chair to steady yourself then shift all your weight onto your left foot, keeping your torso erect and spine tall. Lift your right leg forward (out in front of your body) as you point the toe. Lift your foot anywhere from 1 to 12 inches off the floor (the higher you lift the leg the more difficult the movement). Drop your foot down to the floor and lightly touch the toe on the ground then lift it again. Repeat for 10 seconds then switch sides.

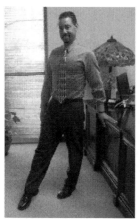 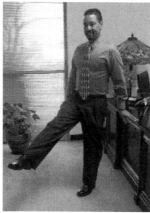

Energizing Movements

Lifting the Sky

Bring your hands up in front of your hips, palms facing up as if you were supporting a large belly in front of you. Slowly pull your palms up towards your chin, keeping your hands a few inches away from the front of your body. When your hands reach your chest rotate the palms down, forward and up until your palms face the sky, and press upward until your arms are extended overhead as if lifting the sky. When your arms are fully extended overhead allow them to swing outward in a wide arc to your sides coming slowly back to the original position.

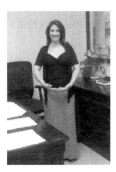 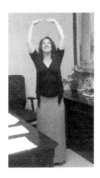

Shake Illness from the Body

Begin in a standing position, feet hip distance apart, arms hanging at the sides of the body. Lift up onto your toes as high as you can and pause. Drop down heavily on the soles of your feet and shake the body and arms vigorously (if this brings you pain simply drop down gently, minimizing the bang at the bottom). Repeat 3 to 4 times.

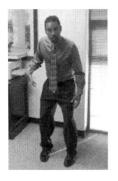 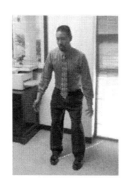

Awakening the Chi

From a standing position with your feet hip distance apart, bend your knees slightly. Inhale deeply through your nose then slowly exhale out through your mouth. Continue to breathe like this the entire time you do the rest of the movements. Take your hands and begin to slap the fronts of your thighs vigorously. You should feel the area being slapped begin to feel tingly; if it hurts, you're slapping too hard. Move to the backs of the thighs, then up to the buttocks. Move up the body slapping the fronts of the hips, belly, chest, shoulders, arms and finally the face.

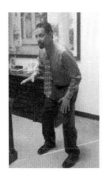 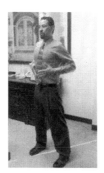

Opening the Door

Stand with your feet slightly wider than hip distance apart. Bend your knees slightly (the deeper you bend your knees the more challenging this movement becomes). Now tuck your tailbone under your spine, lengthening the lower back. Let your arms dangle at your sides. Roll your shoulders gently open and relax the chest. Allow your head to float off your shoulders. Inhale deeply through your nose as you slowly raise your arms in front of you, palms facing down towards the ground, muscles relaxed and soft until your arms reach shoulder height. Raise your palms so that they face forward and exhale through your mouth as you slowly lower your arms back down to their original position. Repeat 5 times.

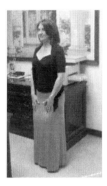 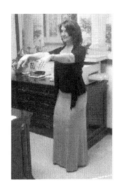

Two Full Moons

Stand with your feet slightly wider than hip distance apart. Bend your knees slightly (the deeper you bend your knees the more challenging this exercise becomes). Now tuck your tailbone under your spine, lengthening the lower back. Let your arms dangle at your sides. Roll your shoulders gently open and relax the chest. Allow your head to float off your shoulders. Inhale deeply through your nose as you slowly raise your arms in front of you, palms facing down towards the ground, muscles relaxed and soft until your arms are up over your head. Swing both arms out to your sides as you exhale and lower your arms back down to your sides. Repeat 5 times.

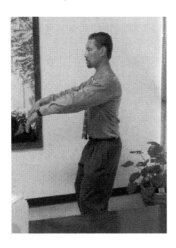 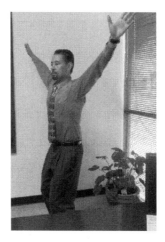

Swimming on Land

Stand with your feet slightly wider than hip distance apart. Bend your knees slightly (the deeper you bend your knees the more challenging this exercise becomes). Now tuck your tailbone under your spine, lengthening the lower back. Bring your hands up in front of your chest, elbows pointing outward. Start to move your hands as if you were doing the breast stroke (a wide circular motion at chest height). Inhale deeply through your nose and exhale slowly through your mouth as you continue to "swim" with your arms. Do this for 5 breaths.

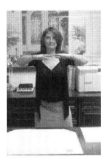 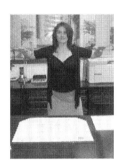

Bending Backwards

Stand with your feet slightly wider than hip distance apart. Now tuck your tailbone under your spine, lengthening the lower back. Place both hands behind you at the small of your back and gently lean backwards. As you begin to lean back, bend your knees slightly and press your hips forward. Allow your chest to rise upward as you look up at the ceiling. Hold for 1 to 2 seconds and return to the starting position. Repeat 5 times.

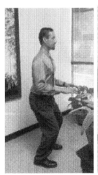 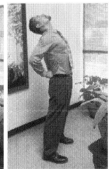

Bending to the sides

Stand with your feet slightly wider than hip distance apart. Place your right hand on your right hip. Bring your left hand up over your head as you gently lean to the right, pressing your left hip out to the left. Reach with your left hand over your head until you feel a gentle stretch all along your left side. Hold for 5 to 10 seconds then switch sides.

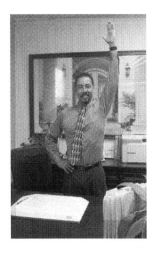 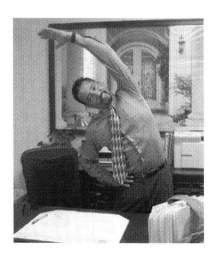

Looking back at the moon

Stand with your feet slightly wider than hip distance apart facing forward. Place both hands on your hips and slowly twist at the waist as you turn your entire upper body to the left. Be sure to keep your feet firmly planted on the floor. Turn your head to the left as if looking behind you and hold for 5 seconds. Switch sides.

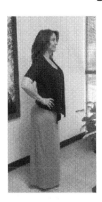 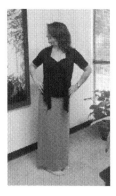

Bellows Breath

The Bellows Breath is adapted from a yogic breathing technique. Its aim is to raise vital energy and increase alertness.

- Inhale and exhale rapidly through your nose, keeping your mouth closed but relaxed. Your breaths in and out should be equal in duration, but as short as possible. This is a noisy breathing exercise.
- Try for 3 in-and-out breath cycles per second. This produces a quick movement of the diaphragm, suggesting a bellows. Breathe normally after each cycle.
- Do not do for more than 15 seconds on your first try. Each time you practice the Bellows Breath, you can increase your time by 5 seconds or so, until you reach a full minute.

If done properly, you may feel invigorated, comparable to the heightened awareness you feel after a good workout. You should feel the effort at the back of the neck, the diaphragm, the chest and the abdomen. Try this breathing exercise the next time you need an energy boost and feel yourself reaching for a cup of coffee. (From Dr. Andrew Weil's website www.drweil.com)

Alternate Nostril Breathing

Alternate nostril breathing creates optimum function of both sides of the brain, improves mood, strengthens the lungs and energizes the body.

- Close off the right nostril with your right thumb then inhale through the left nostril to a three-count
- Hold your breath for an eight-count
- Release your thumb from your right nostril and exhale through the right nostril for a count of 6 as you close off the left nostril with your left thumb.

- Now inhale through your right nostril for a three-count and repeat this on both sides for 1 to 3 minutes.

4-7-8 Breath

This exercise is utterly simple, takes almost no time, requires no equipment and can be done anywhere. Although you can do the exercise in any position, it is best to sit with your back straight while learning the exercise. Place the tip of your tongue against the ridge of tissue just behind your upper front teeth, and keep it there through the entire exercise. You will be exhaling through your mouth around your tongue; try pursing your lips slightly if this seems awkward.

- Exhale completely through your mouth, making a whoosh sound.
- Close your mouth and inhale quietly through your nose to a mental count of **4**.
- Hold your breath for a count of **7**.
- Exhale completely through your mouth, making a whoosh sound to a count of **8**.

This is 1 breath. Now inhale again and repeat the cycle 3 more times for a total of 4 breaths. (From Dr. Andrew Weil's website www.drweil.com)

Cooling breath

This breath is meant to cool the nervous system and mind. This simple breathing technique is a great way to relieve stress and cool down a hot temper.

- Stick your tongue out of your mouth and curl it creating a small "straw-" like tube with the tongue.
- Slowly and smoothly suck air in through the tongue filling the lungs with air. Draw the tongue into the mouth and close the lips.

- Hold the breath for a count of 5, then exhale slowly and smoothly through the nostrils.
- Repeat 3 times.

Strength Movements

A note on breathing during the strength movements: Try to exhale during the harder phase of each movement and inhale during the easier part of each movement.

Pulling the Bow

Stand with your feet slightly wider than hip distance apart. Swing your elbows outward as you bring your hands up to your chest, palms facing the body. Ball your hands into fists (tops of the fists should be facing one another). The next movement is like an archer pulling his bow: keeping the left hand where it is, slowly extend your right arm out to the right side at shoulder height as if ready to the shoot the arrow. Hold for a moment feeling the tension between the bow and the string. Slowly bring your right hand back to your chest. Keep the right hand were it is and slowly extend your left arm out to the left side at shoulder height as if ready to shoot the arrow. Hold for a moment feeling the tension between the bow and the string. Slowly bring the left hand back to your chest.

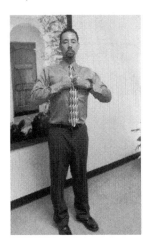 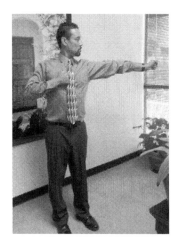

Punch with Eye Glaring

Stand with your feet slightly wider than hip distance apart. Making sure that your tailbone is tucked under, bring your hands up so that your hands and wrists are in line with your elbows, palms facing up, elbows pressed against your ribcage. Ball your fists and draw the elbows back until your wrists are pressed against your ribcage. Give me your best Kung Fu glare as you punch with your right hand, slowly rotating the hand so that the palm faces the ground, moving slowly like you were punching in mud. Pull your hand back and repeat with the left hand. Repeat 3 to 4 times.

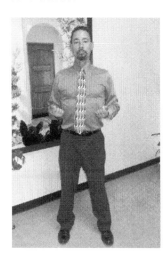 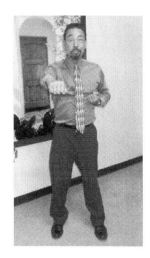

Chair Squats

Begin by sitting on a chair with feet hip distance apart. Your knees should be aligned directly over your ankles. Sit up tall and bring your arms out in front of you at shoulder height with the palms of your hands pointed in towards the center line of your body. Stand, then drop the buttocks down as if to sit, trying to keep as much weight *off* the chair as you can when coming down to the seated position. Press back up to the original position. Repeat 10 times.

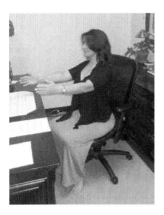 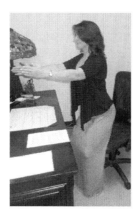

Chair Dips

Sit on an immovable chair or desk. Place your hands on either side of your hips with your palms flat on the desk or seat of the chair and your fingers pointed forward. With your feet on the floor, walk your feet as far away from you as you can, sliding your buttocks off the edge of the chair or desk. After your buttocks have cleared the edge of the chair or desk and are hovering off the ground, your body supported by your arms and feet, you can keep your knees bent and aligned over the ankles. If you would like a little more of a challenge, you can extend your legs and balance on your heels. Keeping the core engaged and the butt lifted, lower your body down towards the ground then press back up to the original starting position. Repeat for 10 seconds.

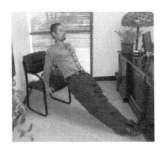 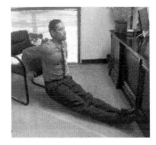

Incline Push-Ups

Stand 3 to 4 feet from a desk or wall. Bring yourself into push-up position with your hands on the desk or wall and your feet on the floor. Hands should be directly below the shoulders and the spine should be long, making sure that your hips don't sag or your bottom isn't sticking up in the air; your body should be angled from the ground to the desk. From this position, lower your chest down to the desk then press back up to your original position. Repeat for 10 seconds.

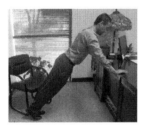 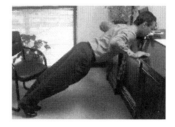

Leg Pull-Downs

Sitting down on an immoveable chair or desk, place your hands on either side of your hips, palms flat on the chair or desk with fingers pointed in front of you. Walk your feet as far away from you as you can, sliding your buttocks off the edge of the chair or desk. After your buttocks has cleared the edge of the chair or desk and are hovering off the ground with your body weight supported by your arms, extend the legs and balance on the heels. Keeping the core engaged and the butt lifted, press your left heel firmly into the ground and lift your right foot as high as you can and hold it up. Bring your right foot back down and then press your right heel firmly into the ground and lift your left foot as high as you can and hold it. Bring your left foot down. Repeat on both sides 10 times.

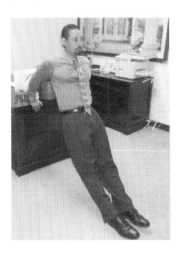
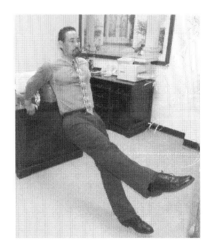

Wide Leg Turnout Squat

Stand with your arms folded at your chest. Spread your legs so they are twice hip distance apart with toes pointed outward at a 45-degree angle from the mid-line of the body. Bend your knees as you drop your buttocks down towards the floor as if you were going to sit in a chair, but be sure to keep your torso as upright as possible. Then return to the starting position. Repeat 10 times.

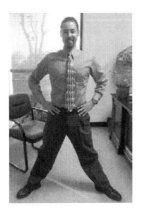
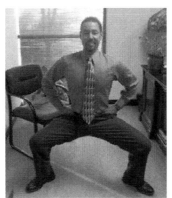

Lunge

Stand with your feet slightly wider than hip distance apart. Place both hands on your hips. Step forward with your right foot approximately 18 to 24 inches. Bend your left knee and slowly kneel until the left knee touches or almost touches the floor. Be sure to keep the torso upright and the spine long. Keeping your feet where they are, slowly stand, then lower the left knee back to the floor. Repeat 10 times then switch sides.

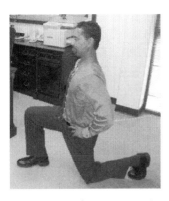
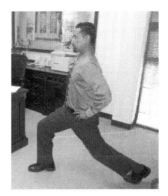

Lateral Raises

Stand with your feet slightly wider than hip distance apart. Drop your arms down to your sides. Keeping your arms long and straight raise them until they reach shoulder height then lower them back to your sides. Repeat 10 times.

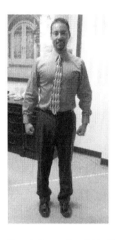 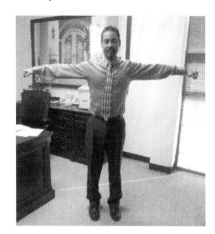

Pushing the Wall

Stand facing a wall that has no furniture in front of it and has no pictures that will interfere with you leaning into it. Rest both hands on the wall at chest height. Bend your elbows slightly. Step back as far as you can with your right foot then press into the wall firmly. Continue to press into the wall for 10 seconds. Switch legs and repeat.

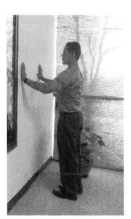 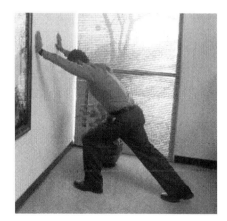

Static Chest Press

This movement can be done either standing or seated. Bring the palms of both hands together in front of your chest. Press your hands together as hard as you can and continue to press them together for 10 seconds. Take your arms down to your sides then swing the arms in big circles a few times

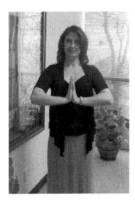

The next 3 movements can be done empty-handed or you can add hand weights, canned goods, full water bottles, etc.

Bicep Curls

Stand with your feet slightly wider than hip distance apart. Drop your arms down to your sides, keeping your elbows against your rib cage. With palms facing forward, bring your hands up to shoulder height then lower down again, doing classic bicep curls for 1 minute.

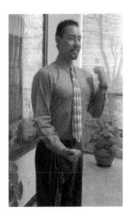
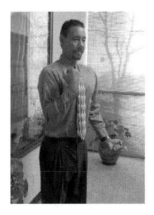

Shoulder Press

Stand with your feet slightly wider than hip distance apart. Take your arms out to the sides and bend your elbows. Hands should come to just above the shoulders and the palms should be facing upward as if supporting a tray in each hand. Press your hands up until your arms are completely extended, then lower back down to complete the shoulder press. Do this for 1 minute.

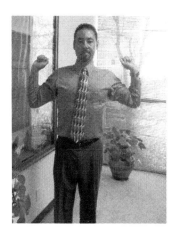 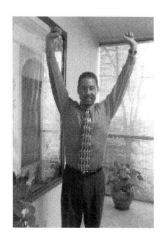

One Minute Activity Segments

Willow Bends in the Wind (Flexibility Focused)

Chair-Supported Downward Facing Dog

Rise from your seated position and walk behind your chair. Secure the chair so that it will not move or roll away. Facing the back of the chair, grab the top of the chair back and then take a step or two backwards away from the chair until your arms are fully extended. Hinge at the hips and lean forward, bringing the torso parallel to the floor beneath you. You should feel a gentle stretch in the low back and hamstring muscles. Hold for 15 seconds.

Bending to the Sides

Stand with your feet slightly wider than hip distance apart. Place your right hand on your right hip. Bring your left hand up over your head as you gently lean to the right, pressing your left hip out to the left. Reach with your left hand over your head until you feel a gentle stretch all along your left side. Hold for 5 to 10 seconds then switch sides.

The Archway

Begin by standing in front of a stable desk or chair. Turn your back to the desk or chair and place the palms of your hands on the desk or chair behind you with your fingers pointed away from your body. Keeping your hands on the desk or chair, take a short step away with both feet, then arch your back and press your chest up towards the ceiling. Gently drop your head back and look up at the ceiling. Hold for 10 seconds and then walk your feet back to the original position.

Curling Serpent (Flexibility Focused)

Seated Forward Fold

Begin in a tall seated position with your feet about hip distance apart Hinge at the hips as you lean forward from the waist. Drape the front of your torso over the front of your thighs, dropping your head between your knees, and grab hold of your ankles. Let your head drop and dangle, relaxing your neck. Pull your lower spine away from your hips. You should feel a gentle stretch in your lower- and mid-back. Hold for 15 seconds and return to your tall seated position.

Seated Twist

Begin in a seated position. With both feet on the floor, gently turn to the right, keeping your spine long yet relaxed. With your right arm, reach to the back of your chair as you twist the torso, using the back of the chair as leverage. Without straining your neck, turn your head and torso as if you were going to look behind you. Hold for 10 seconds. Repeat on the opposite side. Return to your tall seated position.

Shake Illness from the Body

Begin in a standing position, feet hip distance apart, arms hanging at the sides of your body. Lift up onto your toes as high as you can and pause. Drop down heavily on the soles of your feet and shake the body and arms vigorously (if this brings you pain simply drop down gently, minimizing the bang at the bottom) and repeat 3 to 4 times.

Flowing River (Flexibility Focused)

Round and Open

Sitting in a chair with your feet on the floor, begin by bringing your shoulders directly above your hips, lengthening your spine upward as your head floats away from your shoulders. Drop your chin down to your chest and slowly lean forward as you roll the shoulders in towards the chest, making an exaggerated hump in your back. Bring your forearms to the fronts of your thighs as you pull the shoulder blades apart. Hold for 15 seconds as you breathe.

Now, slowly, one vertebra at a time, bring yourself back up to a tall seated position then roll the shoulders back, open the chest, arch the back and look up to the ceiling. Breathe deeply as you let your arms drop down to your sides. Hold for 15 seconds and come back to the tall seated position.

Standing Single Leg Circles

Stand with your feet hip distance apart with your desk or a chair that will not move directly to your left. Place your left hand on your desk or chair to steady yourself then shift all your weight onto your left foot, keeping your torso erect and spine tall. Lift your right leg out to the side pointing your toe at the floor (your foot should be about 6 inches off the floor). Make a circle with your foot about the size of a volley ball for 15 seconds. Switch sides.

Hip Swivels

Stand with your feet hip distance apart. Place your hands on your hips and slowly start to roll your hips in a circle. With each swivel of your hips make the circles a little bigger. After 10 seconds, switch directions.

Swaying Palm (Flexibility Focused)

Bending to the sides

Stand with your feet slightly wider than hip distance apart. Place your right hand on your right hip. Bring your left hand up over your head as you gently lean to the right, pressing your left hip out to the left. Reach with your left hand over your head until you feel a gentle stretch all along your left side. Hold for 10 seconds then switch sides.

Bending Backwards

Stand with your feet slightly wider than hip distance apart. Now tuck your tailbone under your spine, lengthening the lower back. Place both hands behind you at the small of your back and gently lean backwards. As you begin to lean back, bend your knees slightly and press your hips forward. Allow your chest to rise upward as you look up at the ceiling. Hold for 15 seconds and return to the starting position.

Lunge

Stand with your feet slightly wider than hip distance apart. Place both hands on your hips. Step forward with your right foot approximately 18 to 24 inches. Bend your left knee and slowly kneel until the left knee touches or almost touches the floor. Be sure to keep your torso upright and your spine long. Keeping your feet where they are, slowly stand, then lower the left knee back to the floor. Repeat 10 times then switch sides.

Supple Leaf (Flexibility Focused)

Turning the Head

Begin in a standing position with arms hanging at your sides and palms of your hands facing your body. *Very slowly* turn your head to the right and look over your right shoulder as you rotate the palms of your hands out so that they point out and away from your body. *Very slowly* turn your head back so that you are looking forward again as you rotate the palms back so that they face your body again. *Very slowly* turn your head to the left and look over your left shoulder as you rotate the palms out so that they point out and away from your body. *Very slowly* turn your head back so that you are looking forward again as you rotate the palms back so that they face your body again. Do this 5 times on each side.

Pec (pectoral) Stretch

From a standing position bring both hands together behind your back and interlace the fingers. Press your chest out as you lift the joined hands upward towards the backs of your shoulders. Hold for 15 seconds.

Quad & Hip Flexor Stretch

Stand and hold onto a chair or your desk with your left hand. Bend your right knee, bringing your right heel up towards your buttocks. Reach down and grab your right ankle. Pull your knee cap down towards the floor and press your right hip gently forward. Hold for 15 seconds. Switch sides.

The Tides (Flexibility Focused)

Chair Squats

Begin by sitting on a chair with feet hip distance apart, knees aligned directly over the ankles. Sit up tall and bring your arms out in front of you at shoulder height with the palms of your hands pointed in towards the centerline of the body. Stand, then drop the buttocks down as if to sit, trying to keep as much weight *off* the chair as you can when coming down to the seated position. Press back up to the original position. Repeat 10 times.

Sitting Man-Style

Begin in a tall seated position. Cross your right ankle over your left knee, creating a triangle shape with your right leg, then gently press down on the inside of your right knee until you feel a gentle stretch through the hip and buttocks. Hold for 15 seconds. Now gently lean forward, bringing the chest down towards the legs; this should intensify the stretch. Hold for another 15 seconds. Switch sides and repeat on the other side, then return to your tall seated position.

Half Eagle

You can do this one from either the standing or seated position. Bring your left arm directly out in front of you at chest level. Bend your elbow and point your forearm and hand up towards the sky. Take your right arm and cross the right bicep under your left elbow as you reach with the right hand up and around the left forearm, grabbing the inside of the left wrist. Hold for 5 to 10 seconds then switch sides.

Awakening Cat (Flexibility Focused)

Round and Open

Sitting in a chair with your feet on the floor, begin by bringing your shoulders directly above your hips, lengthening your spine upward as your head floats away from your shoulders. Drop your chin down to your chest and slowly lean forward as you roll the shoulders in towards the chest, making an exaggerated hump in your back. Bring your forearms to the fronts of your thighs as you pull your shoulder blades apart. Hold for 15 seconds as you breathe.

Now, slowly, one vertebra at a time, bring yourself back up to a tall seated position, then roll your shoulders back, open your chest, arch your back and look up to the ceiling. Let your arms drop down to the sides and breathe deeply. Hold for fifteen seconds and come back to the tall seated position.

Incline Push-Ups

Stand 3 to 4 feet from a desk or wall. Bring yourself into push-up position with your hands on the desk or wall and your feet on the floor. Hands should be directly below the shoulders and the spine should be long, making sure that your hips don't sag or your bottom isn't sticking up in the air; your body should be angled from the ground to the desk. From this position, lower your chest down to the desk then press back up to your original position. Repeat for 10 seconds.

Opening the Door

Stand with your feet slightly wider than hip distance apart. Bend your knees slightly (the deeper you bend your knees the more challenging this movement becomes). Now tuck your tailbone under your spine, lengthening the lower back. Let your arms dangle at your sides. Roll your shoulders gently open and relax your chest. Allow your head to float off your shoulders. Inhale deeply through your nose as you slowly raise your arms in front of you, palms facing down towards the ground, muscles relaxed and soft until your arms reach shoulder height. Raise your palms so that they face forward and exhale through your mouth as you slowly lower your arms back down to their original position. Repeat 5 times.

Monkey in the Tree (Flexibility Focused)

Neck Rolls

Stand with your feet hip distance apart, arms hanging down to your sides. Gently roll your head in small circles and then slowly make each circle a little bigger. After 5 or 10 seconds, reverse the direction of your circles.

Awakening the Chi

From a standing position with feet hip distance apart bend your knees slightly. Inhale deeply through your nose then slowly exhale out through your mouth. Continue to breathe like this the entire time you do the rest of the movements. Take your hands and begin to slap the fronts of your thighs vigorously. You should feel the area being slapped begin to feel tingly; if it hurts, you're slapping too hard. Move to the backs of your thighs, then up to the buttocks. Move up the body slapping the fronts of your hips, belly, chest, shoulders, arms and finally the face. This should take about 30 seconds.

Triceps Stretch

You can do this one from either the standing or seated position. Reach up towards the ceiling with your right arm then drop your right hand down behind your head, pointing your right elbow up towards the ceiling. Reach up to your right elbow with your left hand and gently pull the elbow towards the midline of your body until you feel a gentle stretch in the back of your right triceps. Hold for 5 to 10 seconds then switch arms.

Hunting Tiger (Strength Focused)

Pulling the Bow

Stand with your feet slightly wider than hip distance apart. Swing your elbows outward as you bring your hands up to your chest, palms facing your body. Ball your hands into fists (tops of the fists should be facing one another). The next movement is like an archer pulling his bow: keep the left hand where it is and slowly extend your right arm out to the right side at shoulder height as if ready to the shoot the arrow. Hold for a moment, feeling the tension between the bow and the string. Slowly bring your right hand back to your chest. Keep the right hand were it is and slowly extend your left arm out to the left side at shoulder height as if ready to shoot the arrow. Hold for a moment, feeling the tension between the bow and the string. Slowly bring your left hand back to your chest.

Chair Dips

 Sit on an immovable chair or desk. Place your hands on either side of your hips with your palms flat on the desk or the seat of the chair, fingers pointed forward. With your feet on the floor, walk your feet as far away from you as you can, sliding your buttocks off the edge of the chair or desk. After your buttocks has cleared the edge of the chair or desk and is hovering off the ground, your body supported by your arms and feet, keep the knees bent and aligned over the ankles. If you would like a little more of a challenge you can extend your legs and balance on your heels. Keeping the core engaged and the butt lifted, lower your body down towards the ground, then press back up to original starting position. Repeat for 15 seconds.

Chair Squats

Begin by sitting on the chair with feet hip distance apart, knees aligned directly over your ankles. Sit up tall and bring your arms out in front of you at shoulder height with the palms of your hands pointed in towards the center line of the body. Stand, then drop the buttocks down as if to sit, trying to keep as much weight *off* the chair as you can when coming down to the seated position. Press back up to the original position. Repeat 10 times.

Crashing Thunder (Strength Focused)

Pushing the Wall

Stand facing a clear wall. Rest both hands on the wall at chest height. Bend your elbows slightly. Step back as far as you can with your right foot then press into the wall firmly. Continue to press into the wall for 15 seconds. Switch legs and repeat.

Swimming on Land

Stand with your feet slightly wider than hip distance apart. Bend your knees slightly (the deeper you bend your knees the more challenging this exercise becomes). Now tuck your tailbone under your spine, lengthening the lower back. Bring your hands up in front of your chest, elbows pointing outward. Start to move your hands as if you were doing the breast stroke (a wide circular motion at chest height). Inhale deeply through your nose and exhale slowly through your mouth as you continue to "swim" with your arms. Do this for 5 breaths.

Leg Pull-Downs

Sitting down on an immoveable chair or desk, place your hands on either side of your hips, palms flat on the chair or desk with fingers pointed in front of you. Walk your feet as far away from you as you can, sliding your buttocks off the edge of the chair or desk. After your buttocks has cleared the edge of the chair or desk and are hovering off the ground with your body weight supported by your arms, extend the legs and balance on the heels. Keeping the core engaged and the butt lifted, press your left heel firmly into the ground and lift your right foot as high as you can and hold it up. Bring your right foot back down and then press your right heel firmly into the ground and lift your left foot as high as you can and hold it. Bring your left foot down. Repeat on both sides 10 times.

Brave Warrior (Strength Focused)

Punch with Eye Glaring

Stand with your feet slightly wider than hip distance apart. Making sure that your tailbone is tucked under, bring your hands up so that your hands and wrists are in line with your elbows, palms facing up, elbows pressed against your ribcage. Ball your fists and draw the elbows back until your wrists are pressed against your ribcage. Give me your best Kung Fu glare as you punch with your right hand, slowly rotating the hand so that the palm faces the ground, moving slowly like you were punching in mud. Pull your hand back and repeat with the left hand. Repeat 3 to 4 times.

Wu Chi Stance

Stand with your feet slightly wider than hip distance apart. Bend your knees slightly (the deeper you bend your knees the more challenging this exercise becomes). Now tuck your tailbone under the spine, lengthening the lower back. Let your arms dangle at your sides. Roll your shoulders gently open and relax the chest. Allow your head to float off your shoulders. Hold for 30 seconds.

Static Chest Press

This movement can be done either standing or seated. Bring the palms of both hands together in front of your chest. Press your hands together as hard as you can and continue to press them together for 10 seconds. Take your arms down to your sides then swing the arms in big circles a few times. Repeat Twice.

Mother Bear (Strength Focused)

Incline Push-Ups

Stand 3 to 4 feet from a desk or wall. Bring yourself into pushup position with your hands on the desk or wall, your feet on the floor. Hands should be directly below your shoulders and the spine should be long, making sure that your hips don't sag or your bottom isn't sticking up in the air. Your body should be angled from the ground to the desk. From this position, lower your chest down to the desk, then press back up to your original position. Repeat for 10 seconds.

Standing Single Leg Side Beats

Stand with your feet hip distance apart with your desk or a chair that will not move directly to your left. Place your left hand on your desk or chair to steady yourself then shift all your weight onto your left foot, keeping your torso erect and spine tall. Lift your right leg sideways (out to the right of your body) as you point the toe. Lift your foot anywhere from 1 to 12 inches off the floor (the higher you lift the leg the more difficult the movement). Drop your foot down to the floor and lightly touch the toe on the ground then lift it again. Repeat for 10 seconds then switch sides.

Lateral Raises

Stand with your feet slightly wider than hip distance apart. Drop your arms down to your sides. Keeping your arms long and straight raise them until they reach shoulder height then lower them back to your sides. Repeat 10 times.

Mighty Wind (Strength Focused)

Pushing the Wall

Stand facing a clear wall. Rest both hands on the wall at chest height. Bend your elbows slightly. Step back as far as you can with your right foot then press into the wall firmly. Continue to press into the wall for 10 seconds. Switch legs and repeat.

Two Full Moons

Stand with your feet slightly wider than hip distance apart. Bend your knees slightly (the deeper you bend your knees the more challenging this exercise becomes). Now tuck your tailbone under your spine, lengthening the lower back. Let your arms dangle at your sides. Roll your shoulders gently open and relax the chest. Allow your head to float off your shoulders. Inhale deeply through your nose as you slowly raise your arms in front of you, palms facing down towards the ground, muscles relaxed and soft until your arms are up over your head. Swing both arms out to your sides as you exhale and lower your arms back down to your sides. Repeat 5 times.

Pulling the Bow

Stand with your feet slightly wider than hip distance apart. Swing your elbows outward as you bring your hands up to your chest, palms facing the body. Ball your hands into fists (tops of the fists should be facing one another). The next movement is like an archer pulling his bow: keeping the left hand where it is, slowly extend your right arm out to the right side at shoulder height as if ready to the shoot the arrow. Hold for a moment feeling the tension between the bow and the string. Slowly bring your right hand back to your chest. Keep the right hand were it is and slowly extend your left arm out to the left side at shoulder height as if ready to shoot the arrow. Hold for a moment feeling the tension between the bow and the string. Slowly bring the left hand back to your chest.

Drunken Elephant (Strength Focused)

Lifting the Knee

Stand with your feet hip distance apart. Shift all your weight onto your left foot and slowly lift your right foot off the ground. Bring your knee up slowly until it is even with your hip (thigh should be parallel to the floor), then slowly lower it back down to the floor. Switch legs.

Punch with Eye Glaring

Stand with your feet slightly wider than hip distance apart. Making sure that your tailbone is tucked under, bring your hands up so that your hands and wrists are in line with your elbows, palms facing up, elbows pressed against your ribcage. Ball your fists and draw the elbows back until your wrists are pressed against your ribcage. Give me your best Kung Fu glare as you punch with your right hand, slowly rotating the hand so that the palm faces the ground, moving slowly like you were punching in mud. Pull your hand back and repeat with the left hand. Repeat 3 to 4 times.

Bicep Curls

Stand with your feet slightly wider than hip distance apart. Drop your arms down to your sides, keeping your elbows against your rib cage. With palms facing forward bring your hands up to shoulder height then lower down again, doing classic bicep curls for 15 seconds.

Angry Hippo (Strength Focused)

Wide Leg Turnout Squat

Stand with your arms folded at your chest. Spread your legs so they are twice hip distance apart with toes pointed outward at a 45-degree angle from the mid-line of the body. Bend your knees as you drop your buttocks down towards the floor as if you were going to sit in a chair, but be sure to keep your torso as upright as possible. Then return to the starting position. Repeat 10 times.

Chair Dips

Sit on an immovable chair or desk. Place your hands on either side of your hips with your palms flat on the desk or the seat of the chair, fingers pointed forward. With your feet on the floor, walk your feet as far away from you as you can, sliding your buttocks off the edge of the chair or desk. After your buttocks has cleared the edge of the chair or desk and is hovering off the ground, your body supported by your arms and feet, keep the knees bent and aligned over the ankles. If you would like a little more of a challenge you can extend your legs and balance on your heels. Keeping the core engaged and the butt lifted, lower your body down towards the ground, then press back up to original starting position. Repeat for 15 seconds.

Raising your Internal Temperature

Stand with your feet at hip distance apart. Begin to march in place very slowly raising your right leg to a slow count of 3 then lowering it to a slow count of 3 then do the same with the left foot. Continue alternating for 10 to 20 seconds.

Ancient Mountain (Strength Focused)

Tree Pose (modified)

Stand with your feet hip distance apart. Shift your weight onto your left foot and bring your right foot off the ground. Place the sole of your right foot against the calf of your left leg. Bring the palms of your hands together in prayer position in the middle of your chest then forcefully push them together. Hold for 10 seconds then switch legs.

Shoulder Press

Stand with your feet slightly wider than hip distance apart. Take your arms out to the sides and bend your elbows. Hands should come to just above the shoulders and the palms should be facing upward as if supporting a tray in each hand. Press your hands up until your arms are completely extended, then lower back down to complete the shoulder press. Do this for 15 seconds.

Lifting the Sky

Bring your hands up in front of your hips, palms facing up as if you were supporting a large belly in front of you. Slowly pull your palms up towards your chin, keeping your hands a few inches away from the front of your body. When your hands reach your chest rotate the palms down, forward and up until your palms face the sky, and press upward until your arms are extended overhead as if lifting the sky. When your arms are fully extended overhead allow them to swing outward in a wide arc to your sides coming slowly back to the original position. Repeat for 20 seconds.

The Stork (Balance Focused)

Sumo Step

Stand with legs twice hip width apart. Drop the buttocks down six to 10 inches bringing you into a wide legged squat position (the deeper the squat the more challenging this becomes). Shift your weight over to your right foot and slowly lift your left foot off the ground 1 to 8 inches. Hold for a count of 5 then slowly lower the left foot back to the ground. Repeat on the opposite side. Repeat entire exercise 3 times.

Baby Camel Prays to the Gods

From a standing position place your hands on the front of your thighs for support, then lean forward as you roll your shoulders inward and round the back, dropping your chin down to your chest creating a humped back. Pause for a moment, and then one vertebra at a time bring yourself back up to your standing position bringing your arms down to your sides. Slowly roll your shoulders back, lift the chest and look to the sky. Repeat 3 times.

Standing Single Leg Side Beats

Stand with your feet hip distance apart with your desk or a chair that will not move directly to your left. Place your left hand on your desk or chair to steady yourself then shift all your weight onto your left foot, keeping your torso erect and spine tall. Lift your right leg sideways (out to the right of your body) as you point the toe. Lift your foot anywhere from 1 to 12 inches off the floor (the higher you lift the leg the more difficult the movement). Drop your foot down to the floor and lightly touch the toe on the ground then lift it again. Repeat for 10 seconds then switch sides.

Ninja on the Roof (Balance Focused)

Wu Chi Stance

Stand with your feet slightly wider than hip distance apart. Bend your knees slightly (the deeper you bend your knees the more challenging this exercise becomes). Now tuck your tailbone under the spine, lengthening the lower back. Let your arms dangle at your sides. Roll your shoulders gently open and relax the chest. Allow your head to float off your shoulders. Hold for 30 seconds.

Empty Step

Stand with your feet hip distance apart. Shift all of your weight onto your left foot and slowly lift your right foot off the ground. Bring your knee up slowly until it is even with your hip. Extend your right foot and bend your left knee, touching the toe of your right foot on the floor about 12 inches in front of you, putting no weight on the right foot (as if you were testing the temperature of the water in a lake you were thinking of swimming in). Lift the knee back up to hip level then return to your starting position. Switch legs.

Mountain Goat on the Ridge (Balance Focused)

Raising your Internal Temperature

Stand with your feet at hip distance apart. Begin to march in place very slowly raising your right leg to a slow count of 3 then lowering it to a slow count of 3 then do the same with the left foot. Continue alternating for 10 to 20 seconds.

Standing Single Leg Front Beats

Stand with your feet at hip distance apart with your desk or a chair that will not move directly to your left. Place your left hand on your desk or chair to steady yourself then shift all your weight onto your left foot, keeping the torso erect and spine tall. Lift your right leg forward (out to in front of your body) as you point the toe. Lift the foot anywhere from one to twelve inches off the floor (the higher you lift the leg the more difficult the movement). Drop the foot down to the floor and lightly touch the toe on the ground then lift it again. Repeat for 10 seconds then switch sides.

Ankle Circles

Stand with your feet hip distance apart. Shift all of your weight onto your left foot and slowly lift your right foot off the ground. Balance there on your left foot for a breath or two then slowly roll the right foot in a circle for 10 seconds. Slowly bring the right foot back down to the ground and repeat with the left foot.

The Flamingo (Balance Focused)

Standing Single Leg Circles

Stand with your feet at hip distance apart with your desk or a chair that will not move directly to your left. Place your left hand on your desk or chair to steady yourself then shift all your weight onto your left foot, keeping your torso erect and spine tall. Lift your right leg out to the side pointing your toe at the floor (your foot should be about six inches off the floor). Make a circle with your foot about the size of a volleyball for 10 seconds. Switch sides.

Standing Single Leg Front Beats

Stand with your feet hip distance apart with your desk or a chair that will not move directly to your left. Place your left hand on your desk or chair to steady yourself then shift all your weight onto your left foot, keeping your torso erect and spine tall. Lift your right leg forward (out in front of your body) as you point the toe. Lift your foot anywhere from 1 to 12 inches off the floor (the higher you lift the leg the more difficult the movement). Drop your foot down to the floor and lightly touch the toe on the ground then lift it again. Repeat for 10 seconds then switch sides.

Standing Single Leg Back Beats

Stand with your feet hip distance apart with your desk or a chair that will not move directly to your left. Place your left hand on your desk or chair to steady yourself then shift all your weight onto your left foot, keeping your torso erect and spine tall. Lift your right leg backwards as you point the toe. Lift your foot anywhere from 1 to 12 inches off the floor (the higher you lift the leg the more difficult the movement). Drop your foot down to the floor and lightly touch the toe on the ground then lift it again. Repeat for 10 seconds then switch sides.

Boulder on a Ridge (Balance Focused)

The Archway

Begin by standing in front of a stable desk or chair. Turn your back to the desk or chair and place the palms of your hands on the desk or chair behind you with your fingers pointed away from your body. Keeping your hands on the desk or chair, take a short step away with both feet, then arch your back and press your chest up towards the ceiling. Gently drop your head back and look up at the ceiling. Hold for 20 seconds and then walk your feet back to the original position.

Modified Hanging Pose

Begin in a standing position with feet hip distance apart. Bend both knees slightly, then lean forward and slowly lower your head as you begin to reach down toward your mid-thighs or knees depending on what feels comfortable for you. Support the upper body with your hands, and allow the spine to lengthen toward the floor as much as feels comfortable. Hold this pose for 5 long, slow, deep breaths.

Yin/Yang (Balance Focused)

Tree Pose (modified)

Stand with your feet hip distance apart. Shift your weight onto your left foot and bring your right foot off the ground. Place the sole of your right foot against the calf of your left leg. Bring the palms of your hands together in prayer position in the middle of your chest then forcefully push them together. Hold for 10 seconds then switch legs.

Bending to the sides

Stand with your feet slightly wider than hip distance apart. Place your right hand on your right hip. Bring your left hand up over your head as you gently lean to the right, pressing your left hip out to the left. Reach with your left hand over your head until you feel a gentle stretch all along your left side. Hold for 5 to 10 seconds then switch sides.

Wu Chi Stance

Stand with your feet slightly wider than hip distance apart. Bend your knees slightly (the deeper you bend your knees the more challenging this exercise becomes). Now tuck your tailbone under the spine, lengthening the lower back. Let your arms dangle at your sides. Roll your shoulders gently open and relax the chest. Allow your head to float off your shoulders. Hold for 30 seconds.

Cheetah Chases Prey (Energizing Focused)

Opening the Door

Stand with your feet slightly wider than hip distance apart. Bend your knees slightly (the deeper you bend your knees the more challenging this movement becomes). Now tuck your tailbone under your spine, lengthening the lower back. Let your arms dangle at your sides. Roll your shoulders gently open and relax the chest. Allow your head to float off your shoulders. Inhale deeply through your nose as you slowly raise your arms in front of you, palms facing down towards the ground, muscles relaxed and soft until your arms reach shoulder height. Raise your palms so that they face forward and exhale through your mouth as you slowly lower your arms back down to their original position. Repeat 5 times.

Bending Backwards

Stand with your feet slightly wider than hip distance apart. Now tuck your tailbone under your spine, lengthening the lower back. Place both hands behind you at the small of your back and gently lean backwards. As you begin to lean back, bend your knees slightly and press your hips forward. Allow your chest to rise upward as you look up at the ceiling. Hold for 1 to 2 seconds and return to the starting position. Repeat 5 times.

Raising your Internal Temperature

Stand with your feet at hip distance apart. Begin to march in place very slowly raising your right leg to a slow count of 3 then lowering it to a slow count of 3 then do the same with the left foot. Continue alternating for 10 to 20 seconds.

Lightning Bolt Strikes a Tree (Energizing Focused)

Looking back at the moon

Stand with your feet slightly wider than hip distance apart facing forward. Place both hands on your hips and slowly twist at the waist as you turn your entire upper body to the left. Be sure to keep your feet firmly planted on the floor. Turn your head to the left as if looking behind you and hold for 5 seconds. Switch sides.

Lifting the Sky

Bring your hands up in front of your hips, palms facing up as if you were supporting a large belly in front of you. Slowly pull your palms up towards your chin, keeping your hands a few inches away from the front of your body. When your hands reach your chest rotate the palms down, forward and up until your palms face the sky, and press upward until your arms are extended overhead as if lifting the sky. When your arms are fully extended overhead allow them to swing outward in a wide arc to your sides coming slowly back to the original position. Repeat for 30 seconds.

Modified Hanging Pose

Begin in a standing position with feet hip distance apart. Bend both knees slightly, then lean forward and slowly lower your head as you begin to reach down toward your mid-thighs or knees depending on what feels comfortable for you. Support the upper body with your hands, and allow the spine to lengthen toward the floor as much as feels comfortable. Hold this pose for 5 long, slow, deep breaths.

Fast-Running Stream (Energizing Focused)

Shake Illness from the Body

Begin in a standing position, feet hip distance apart, arms hanging at the sides of the body. Lift up onto your toes as high as you can and pause. Drop down heavily on the soles of your feet and shake the body and arms vigorously (if this brings you pain simply drop down gentl0y, minimizing the bang at the bottom). Repeat 3 to 4 times.

Alternate Nostril Breathing

Alternate nostril breathing creates optimum function of both sides of the brain, improves mood, strengthens the lungs and energizes the body.

- Close off the right nostril with your right thumb then inhale through the left nostril to a three-count
- Hold your breath for an eight-count
- Release your thumb from your right nostril and exhale through the right nostril for a count of 6 as you close off the left nostril with your left thumb.

- Now inhale through your right nostril for a three-count and repeat this on both sides a few times.

Swimming on Land

Stand with your feet slightly wider than hip distance apart. Bend your knees slightly (the deeper you bend your knees the more challenging this exercise becomes). Now tuck your tailbone under your spine, lengthening the lower back. Bring your hands up in front of your chest, elbows pointing outward. Start to move your hands as if you were doing the breast stroke (a wide circular motion at chest height). Inhale deeply through your nose and exhale slowly through your mouth as you continue to "swim" with your arms. Do this for 5 breaths.

Happy Toddler (Energizing Focused)

Lifting the Sky

Bring your hands up in front of your hips, palms facing up as if you were supporting a large belly in front of you. Slowly pull your palms up towards your chin, keeping your hands a few inches away from the front of your body. When your hands reach your chest rotate the palms down, forward and up until your palms face the sky, and press upward until your arms are extended overhead as if lifting the sky. When your arms are fully extended overhead allow them to swing outward in a wide arc to your sides coming slowly back to the original position. Repeat for 30 seconds.

Bending to the sides

Stand with your feet slightly wider than hip distance apart. Place your right hand on your right hip. Bring your left hand up over your head as you gently lean to the right, pressing your left hip out to the left. Reach with your left hand over your head until you feel a gentle stretch all along your left side. Hold for 5 to 10 seconds then switch sides.

Looking back at the moon

Stand with your feet slightly wider than hip distance apart facing forward. Place both hands on your hips and slowly twist at the waist as you turn your entire upper body to the left. Be sure to keep your feet firmly planted on the floor. Turn your head to the left as if looking behind you and hold for 5 seconds. Switch sides.

Electric Eel (Energizing Focused)

Bellows Breath

The Bellows Breath is adapted from a yogic breathing technique. Its aim is to raise vital energy and increase alertness.

- Inhale and exhale rapidly through your nose, keeping your mouth closed but relaxed. Your breaths in and out should be equal in duration, but as short as possible. This is a noisy breathing exercise.
- Try for 3 in-and-out breath cycles per second. This produces a quick movement of the diaphragm, suggesting a bellows. Breathe normally after each cycle.

Shake Illness from the Body

Begin in a standing position, feet hip distance apart, arms hanging at the sides of the body. Lift up onto your toes as high as you can and pause. Drop down heavily on the soles of your feet and shake the body and arms vigorously (if this brings you pain simply drop down gentl0y, minimizing the bang at the bottom). Repeat 3 to 4 times.

Hip Swivels

Stand with your feet hip distance apart. Place your hands on your hips and slowly start to roll your hips in a circle. With each swivel of your hips make the circles a little bigger. After 10 seconds, switch directions.

Spicy Dish (Energizing Focused)

Swimming on Land

Stand with your feet slightly wider than hip distance apart. Bend your knees slightly (the deeper you bend your knees the more challenging this exercise becomes). Now tuck your tailbone under your spine, lengthening the lower back. Bring your hands up in front of your chest, elbows pointing outward. Start to move your hands as if you were doing the breast stroke (a wide circular motion at chest height). Inhale deeply through your nose and exhale slowly through your mouth as you continue to "swim" with your arms. Do this for 5 breaths.

Bending Backwards

Stand with your feet slightly wider than hip distance apart. Now tuck your tailbone under your spine, lengthening the lower back. Place both hands behind you at the small of your back and gently lean backwards. As you begin to lean back, bend your knees slightly and press your hips forward. Allow your chest to rise upward as you look up at the ceiling. Hold for 1 to 2 seconds and return to the starting position. Repeat 5 times.

Bending to the sides

Stand with your feet slightly wider than hip distance apart. Place your right hand on your right hip. Bring your left hand up over your head as you gently lean to the right, pressing your left hip out to the left. Reach with your left hand over your head until you feel a gentle stretch all along your left side. Hold for 5 to 10 seconds then switch sides.

Three Minute Activity Segments

Shifting Sand (Flexibility Focused)

Round and Open

Sitting in a chair with your feet on the floor, begin by bringing your shoulders directly above your hips, lengthening your spine upward as your head floats away from your shoulders. Drop your chin down to your chest and slowly lean forward as you roll the shoulders in towards the chest, making an exaggerated hump in your back. Bring your forearms to the fronts of your thighs as you pull the shoulder blades apart. Hold for 30 seconds as you breathe.

Now, slowly, one vertebra at a time, bring yourself back up to a tall seated position then roll the shoulders back, open the chest, arch the back and look up to the ceiling. Breathe deeply as you let your arms drop down to your sides. Hold for 30 seconds and come back to the tall seated position.

Cross Legged Seated Twist

Begin in a tall seated position. Cross your right leg tightly over the left as if you were wearing a short skirt or kilt. Gently turn to the right, keeping your spine long yet relaxed. With your right arm reach to the back of your chair as you twist the torso, using the back of the chair as leverage. With your left hand gently press your knees towards the left side of the chair. Without straining your neck, turn your head and torso as if you were going to look behind you. Hold for 30 seconds. Repeat on the opposite side. Return to the tall seated position.

Lifting the Knee

Stand with your feet hip distance apart. Shift all your weight onto your left foot and slowly lift your right foot off the ground. Bring your knee up slowly until it is even with your hip (thigh should be parallel to the floor), then slowly lower it back down to the floor. Switch legs.

Modified Hanging Pose

Begin in a standing position with feet hip distance apart. Bend both knees slightly, then lean forward and slowly lower your head as you begin to reach down toward your mid-thighs or knees depending on what feels comfortable for you. Support the upper body with your hands, and allow the spine to lengthen toward the floor as much as feels comfortable. Hold this pose for 5 long, slow, deep breaths.

Placid Lake (Flexibility Focused)

Seated Twist

Begin in a tall seated position. With both feet on the floor, gently turn to the right keeping your spine long, yet relaxed. With your right arm, reach to the back of your chair as you twist the torso using the back of the chair as leverage. Without straining your neck, turn your head and torso as if you were going to look behind you. Hold for 30 seconds. Repeat on the opposite side. Return to your tall seated position.

Half Eagle

You can do this one from either the standing or seated position. Bring your left arm directly out in front of you at chest level, bend the elbow and point your forearm and hand up towards the sky. Take your right arm and cross the right bicep under your left elbow as you reach with your right hand up and around your left forearm grabbing the inside of the left wrist. Hold for 15 seconds then switch sides.

Punch with Eye Glaring

Stand with your feet slightly wider than hip distance apart. Making sure that your tailbone is tucked under, bring your hands up so that your hands and wrists are in line with your elbows, palms facing up, elbows pressed against your ribcage. Ball your fists and draw the elbows back until your wrists are pressed against your ribcage. Give me your best Kung Fu glare as you punch with your right hand, slowly rotating the hand so that the palm faces the ground, moving slowly like you were punching in mud. Pull your hand back and repeat with the left hand. Repeat 3 to 4 times.

The Archway

Begin by standing in front of a stable desk or chair. Turn your back to the desk or chair and place the palms of your hands on the desk or chair behind you with your fingers pointed away from your body. Keeping your hands on the desk or chair, take a short step away with both feet, then arch your back and press your chest up towards the ceiling. Gently drop your head back and look up at the ceiling. Hold for 30 seconds and then walk your feet back to the original position.

The Lazy Lion (Flexibility Focused)

Sitting Man-Style

Begin in a tall seated position. Cross your right ankle over your left knee, creating a triangle shape with your right leg, then gently press down on the inside of your right knee until you feel a gentle stretch through the hip and buttocks. Hold for 30 seconds. Now gently lean forward, bringing the chest down towards the legs; this should intensify the stretch. Hold for another 30 seconds. Switch sides and repeat on the other side, then return to your tall seated position.

Static Chest Press

This movement can be done either standing or seated. Bring the palms of both hands together in front of your chest. Press your hands together as hard as you can and continue to press them together for 30 seconds. Take your arms down to your sides then swing the arms in big circles a few times.

Quad & Hip Flexor Stretch

Stand and hold onto a chair or your desk with your left hand. Bend your right knee bringing your right heel up towards your buttocks. Reach down and grab your right ankle. Pull your knee cap down towards the floor and press your right hip gently forward. Hold for five to 10 seconds. Switch sides.

Pec (pectoral) Stretch

From a standing position bring both hands together behind your back and interlace the fingers. Press your chest out as you lift the joined hands upward, towards the backs of your shoulders. Hold for 30 seconds.

Reeds in the Breeze (Flexibility Focused)

Baby Camel Prays to the Gods

From a standing position place your hands on the front of your thighs for support, then lean forward as you roll your shoulders inward and round the back, dropping your chin down to your chest creating a humped back. Pause for a moment, and then one vertebra at a time bring yourself back up to your standing position bringing your arms down to your sides. Slowly roll your shoulders back, lift the chest and look to the sky. Repeat 3 times.

Bending to the sides

Stand with your feet slightly wider than hip distance apart. Place your right hand on your right hip. Bring your left hand up over your head as you gently lean to the right, pressing your left hip out to the left. Reach with your left hand over your head until you feel a gentle stretch all along your left side. Hold for 15 seconds then switch sides.

Hip Swivels

Stand with your feet hip distance apart. Place your hands on your hips and slowly start to roll your hips in a circle. With each swivel of your hips make the circles a little bigger. After 15 seconds, switch directions. Repeat twice.

Two Full Moons

Stand with your feet slightly wider than hip distance apart. Bend your knees slightly (the deeper you bend your knees the more challenging this exercise becomes). Now tuck your tailbone under your spine, lengthening the lower back. Let your arms dangle at your sides. Roll your shoulders gently open and relax the chest. Allow your head to float off your shoulders. Inhale deeply through your nose as you slowly raise your arms in front of you, palms facing down towards the ground, muscles relaxed and soft until your arms are up over your head. Swing both arms out to your sides as you exhale and lower your arms back down to your sides. Repeat 5 times.

Clouds on the Horizon (Flexibility Focused)

Turning the Head

Begin in a standing position with arms hanging at your sides and the palms of your hands facing your body. *Very slowly* turn your head to the right and look over your right shoulder as you rotate the palms of your hands out so that they point out and away from your body. *Very slowly* turn your head back so that you are looking forward again as you rotate your palms back so that they face your body again. *Very slowly* turn your head to the left and look over your left shoulder as you rotate your palms out so that they point out and away from your body. *Very slowly* turn your head back so that you are looking forward again as you rotate your palms back so that they face your body again.

Shoulder Rolls

Stand with your feet hip distance apart, arms hanging down to your sides. Gently roll the shoulders forward, down and back making as big a circle with the shoulders as you comfortably can. After 30 seconds, reverse the direction of your circles.

Ankle Circles

Stand with your feet hip distance apart. Shift all of your weight onto your left foot and slowly lift your right foot off the ground. Balance there on your left foot for a breath or two then slowly roll the right foot in a circle for 10 seconds. Slowly bring the right foot back down to the ground and repeat with the left foot.

Side-Step Lunge

Begin in a standing position with feet hip distance apart. Step with the right foot to the right about 12 inches. Keep the left knee straight and bend the right knee, leaning out towards your right foot until you feel a gentle stretch on the inside of your left leg. Hold for 30 seconds then switch sides.

Deeply Rooted Tree (Flexibility Focused)

Calf Stretch

From a standing position turn and face your desk or wall. Place the palms of your hands on the desk or wall and bend your left knee slightly as you take your right foot and step back. Press your heel down towards the ground and lean gently forward. You should feel a gentle stretch at the back of your lower right leg. Hold for 30 seconds then switch legs.

Seated Forward Fold

Begin in a tall seated position. Bring your feet to about hip distance apart and hinge at the hips as you lean forward from the waist. Drape the front of your torso over the front of your thighs, dropping your head between your knees and grabbing hold of your ankles. Let your head drop and dangle, relaxing your neck. Pull your lower spine away from your hips. You should feel a gentle stretch in your low- and mid-back. Hold for 30 seconds and return to your tall seated position.

Wide Leg Turnout Squat

Stand with your arms folded at your chest. Spread your legs so they are twice hip distance apart with toes pointed outward at a 45-degree angle from the mid-line of the body. Bend your knees as you drop your buttocks down towards the floor as if you were going to sit in a chair, but be sure to keep your torso as upright as possible. Then return to the starting position. Repeat for 1 minute.

Pec (pectoral) Stretch

From a standing position bring both hands together behind your back and interlace the fingers. Press your chest out as you lift the joined hands upward, towards the backs of your shoulders. Hold for 30 seconds.

Young Bull (Strength Focused)

Wide Leg Turnout Squat

Stand with your arms folded at your chest. Spread your legs so they are twice hip distance apart with toes pointed outward at a 45-degree angle from the mid-line of the body. Bend your knees as you drop your buttocks down towards the floor as if you were going to sit in a chair but be sure to keep your torso as upright as possible. Then return to the starting position. Repeat for 1 minute.

Pulling the Bow

Stand with your feet slightly wider than hip distance apart. Swing your elbows outward as you bring your hands up to your chest, palms facing the body. Ball your hands into fists (tops of the fists should be facing one another). The next movement is like an archer pulling his bow: keeping the left hand where it is, slowly extend your right arm out to the right side at shoulder height as if ready to the shoot the arrow. Hold for a moment feeling the tension between the bow and the string. Slowly bring your right hand back to your chest. Keep the right hand were it is and slowly extend your left arm out to the left side at shoulder height as if ready to shoot the arrow. Hold for a moment feeling the tension between the bow and the string. Slowly bring the left hand back to your chest. Repeat twice.

Pushing the Wall

Stand facing a clear wall. Rest both hands on the wall at chest height. Bend your elbows slightly. Step back as far as you can with your right foot then press into the wall firmly. Continue to press into the wall for 30 seconds. Switch legs and repeat.

Chair Dips

Sit on an immovable chair or desk. Place your hands on either side of your hips with your palms flat on the desk or the seat of the chair, fingers pointed forward. With your feet on the floor, walk your feet as far away from you as you can, sliding your buttocks off the edge of the chair or desk. After your buttocks has cleared the edge of the chair or desk and is hovering off the ground, your body supported by your arms and feet, keep the knees bent and aligned over the ankles. If you would like a little more of a challenge you can extend your legs and balance on your heels. Keeping the core engaged and the butt lifted, lower your body down towards the ground, then press back up to original starting position. Repeat for 20 seconds.

Tsunami (Strength Focused)

Wu Chi Stance

Stand with your feet slightly wider than hip distance apart. Bend your knees slightly (the deeper you bend your knees the more challenging this exercise becomes). Now tuck your tailbone under the spine, lengthening the lower back. Let your arms dangle at your sides. Roll your shoulders gently open and relax the chest. Allow your head to float off your shoulders. Hold for 30 seconds.

Lateral Raises

Stand with your feet slightly wider than hip distance apart. Drop your arms down to your sides. Keeping your arms long and straight raise them until they reach shoulder height then lower them back to your sides. Repeat for 30 seconds.

Static Chest Press

This movement can be done either standing or seated. Bring the palms of both hands together in front of your chest. Press your hands together as hard as you can and continue to press them together for 30 seconds. Take your arms down to your sides then swing the arms in big circles a few times.

Standing Single Leg Back Beats

Stand with your feet hip distance apart with your desk or a chair that will not move directly to your left. Place your left hand on your desk or chair to steady yourself then shift all your weight onto your left foot, keeping your torso erect and spine tall. Lift your right leg backwards as you point the toe. Lift your foot anywhere from 1 to 12 inches off the floor (the higher you lift the leg the more difficult the movement). Drop your foot down to the floor and lightly touch the toe on the ground then lift it again. Repeat for 30 seconds then switch sides.

The Plough Horse (Strength Focused)

Leg Pull-Downs

Sitting down on an immoveable chair or desk, place your hands on either side of your hips, palms flat on the chair or desk with fingers pointed in front of you. Walk your feet as far away from you as you can, sliding your buttocks off the edge of the chair or desk. After your buttocks has cleared the edge of the chair or desk and are hovering off the ground with your body weight supported by your arms, extend the legs and balance on the heels. Keeping the core engaged and the butt lifted, press your left heel firmly into the ground and lift your right foot as high as you can and hold it up. Bring your right foot back down and then press your right heel firmly into the ground and lift your left foot as high as you can and hold it. Bring your left foot down. Repeat on both sides 10 times.

Shoulder Press

Stand with your feet slightly wider than hip distance apart. Take your arms out to the sides and bend your elbows. Hands should come to just above the shoulders and the palms should be facing upward as if supporting a tray in each hand. Press your hands up until your arms are completely extended, then lower back down to complete the shoulder press. Do this for 1 minute.

Incline Push-Ups

Stand 3 to 4 feet from a desk or wall. Bring yourself into pushup position with your hands on the desk or wall, your feet on the floor. Hands should be directly below your shoulders and the spine should be long, making sure that your hips don't sag or your bottom isn't sticking up in the air. Your body should be angled from the ground to the desk. From this position, lower your chest down to the desk, then press back up to your original position. Repeat for 30 seconds.

Side-Step Lunge

Begin in a standing position with feet hip distance apart. Step with the right foot to the right about 12 inches. Keep the left knee straight and bend the right knee, leaning out towards your right foot until you feel a gentle stretch on the inside of your left leg. Hold for 30 seconds then switch sides.

Stone Temple (Strength Focused)

Wide Leg Turnout Squat

Stand with your arms folded at your chest. Spread your legs so they are twice hip distance apart with toes pointed outward at a 45-degree angle from the mid-line of the body. Bend your knees as you drop your buttocks down towards the floor as if you were going to sit in a chair but be sure to keep your torso as upright as possible. Then return to the starting position. Repeat for 1 minute.

Punch with Eye Glaring

Stand with your feet slightly wider than hip distance apart. Making sure that your tailbone is tucked under, bring your hands up so that your hands and wrists are in line with your elbows, palms facing up, elbows pressed against your ribcage. Ball your fists and draw the elbows back until your wrists are pressed against your ribcage. Give me your best Kung Fu glare as you punch with your right hand, slowly rotating the hand so that the palm faces the ground, moving slowly like you were punching in mud. Pull your hand back and repeat with the left hand. Repeat 3 to 4 times.

Wu Chi Stance

Stand with your feet slightly wider than hip distance apart. Bend your knees slightly (the deeper you bend your knees the more challenging this exercise becomes). Now tuck your tailbone under the spine, lengthening the lower back. Let your arms dangle at your sides. Roll your shoulders gently open and relax the chest. Allow your head to float off your shoulders. Hold for 60 seconds.

Incline Push-Ups

Stand 3 to 4 feet from a desk or wall. Bring yourself into pushup position with your hands on the desk or wall, your feet on the floor. Hands should be directly below your shoulders and the spine should be long, making sure that your hips don't sag or your bottom isn't sticking up in the air. Your body should be angled from the ground to the desk. From this position, lower your chest down to the desk, then press back up to your original position. Repeat for 30 seconds.

Deep Faith (Strength Focused)

Chair Squats

Begin by sitting on a chair with feet hip distance apart. Your knees should be aligned directly over your ankles. Sit up tall and bring your arms out in front of you at shoulder height with the palms of your hands pointed in towards the center line of your body. Stand, then drop the buttocks down as if to sit, trying to keep as much weight *off* the chair as you can when coming down to the seated position. Press back up to the original position. Repeat for 30 seconds.

Sitting Man-Style

Begin in a tall seated position. Cross your right ankle over your left knee, creating a triangle shape with your right leg, then gently press down on the inside of your right knee until you feel a gentle stretch through the hip and buttocks. Hold for 30 seconds. Now gently lean forward, bringing the chest down towards the legs; this should intensify the stretch. Hold for another 30 seconds. Switch sides and repeat on the other side, then return to your tall seated position.

Half Eagle

You can do this one from either the standing or seated position. Bring your left arm directly out in front of you at chest level, bend the elbow and point your forearm and hand up towards the sky. Take your right arm and cross the right bicep under your left elbow as you reach with your right hand up and around your left forearm grabbing the inside of the left wrist. Hold for30 seconds then switch sides.

Static Chest Press

This movement can be done either standing or seated. Bring the palms of both hands together in front of your chest. Press your hands together as hard as you can and continue to press them together for 30 seconds. Take your arms down to your sides then swing the arms in big circles a few times.

Corner Stone (Strength Focused)

Shoulder Press

Stand with your feet slightly wider than hip distance apart. Take your arms out to the sides and bend your elbows. Hands should come to just above the shoulders and the palms should be facing upward as if supporting a tray in each hand. Press your hands up until your arms are completely extended, then lower back down to complete the shoulder press. Do this for 30 seconds.

Bicep Curls

Stand with your feet slightly wider than hip distance apart. Drop your arms down to your sides, keeping your elbows against your rib cage. With palms facing forward bring your hands up to shoulder height then lower down again, doing classic bicep curls for 30 seconds.

Lunge

Stand with your feet slightly wider than hip distance apart. Place both hands on your hips. Step forward with your right foot approximately 18 to 24 inches. Bend your left knee and slowly kneel until the left knee touches or almost touches the floor. Be sure to keep the torso upright and the spine long. Keeping your feet where they are, slowly stand, then lower the left knee back to the floor. Repeat for 30 seconds then switch sides.

Empty Step

Stand with your feet hip distance apart. Shift all of your weight onto your left foot and slowly lift your right foot off the ground. Bring your knee up slowly until it is even with your hip. Extend your right foot and bend your left knee, touching the toe of your right foot on the floor about 12 inches in front of you, putting no weight on the right foot (as if you were testing the temperature of the water in a lake you were thinking of swimming in). Hold for 30 seconds. Lift the knee back up to hip level then return to your starting position. Switch legs.

Squirrel on a Wire (Balance Focused)

Lifting the Knee

Stand with your feet hip distance apart. Shift all your weight onto your left foot and slowly lift your right foot off the ground. Bring your knee up slowly until it is even with your hip (thigh should be parallel to the floor). Hold it there for 30 seconds then slowly lower it back down to the floor. Switch legs.

Standing Single Leg Side Beats

Stand with your feet hip distance apart with your desk or a chair that will not move directly to your left. Place your left hand on your desk or chair to steady yourself then shift all your weight onto your left foot, keeping your torso erect and spine tall. Lift your right leg sideways (out to the right of your body) as you point the toe. Lift your foot anywhere from 1 to 12 inches off the floor (the higher you lift the leg the more difficult the movement). Drop your foot down to the floor and lightly touch the toe on the ground then lift it again. Repeat for 30 seconds then switch sides.

Opening the Door

Stand with your feet slightly wider than hip distance apart. Bend your knees slightly (the deeper you bend your knees the more challenging this movement becomes). Now tuck your tailbone under your spine, lengthening the lower back. Let your arms dangle at your sides. Roll your shoulders gently open and relax the chest. Allow your head to float off your shoulders. Inhale deeply through your nose as you slowly raise your arms in front of you, palms facing down towards the ground, muscles relaxed and soft until your arms reach shoulder height. Raise your palms so that they face forward and exhale through your mouth as you slowly lower your arms back down to their original position. Repeat 5 times.

Leg Pull-Downs

Sitting down on an immoveable chair or desk, place your hands on either side of your hips, palms flat on the chair or desk with fingers pointed in front of you. Walk your feet as far away from you as you can, sliding your buttocks off the edge of the chair or desk. After your buttocks has cleared the edge of the chair or desk and are hovering off the ground with your body weight supported by your arms, extend the legs and balance on the heels. Keeping the core engaged and the butt lifted, press your left heel firmly into the ground and lift your right foot as high as you can and hold it up. Bring your right foot back down and then press your right heel firmly into the ground and lift your left foot as high as you can and hold it. Bring your left foot down. Repeat on both sides 10 times.

Mother Holding Twins (Balance Focused)

Wu Chi Stance

Stand with your feet slightly wider than hip distance apart. Bend your knees slightly (the deeper you bend your knees the more challenging this exercise becomes). Now tuck your tailbone under the spine, lengthening the lower back. Let your arms dangle at your sides. Roll your shoulders gently open and relax the chest. Allow your head to float off your shoulders. Hold for 30 seconds.

Standing Single Leg Front Beats

Stand with your feet hip distance apart with your desk or a chair that will not move directly to your left. Place your left hand on your desk or chair to steady yourself then shift all your weight onto your left foot, keeping your torso erect and spine tall. Lift your right leg forward (out in front of your body) as you point the toe. Lift your foot anywhere from 1 to 12 inches off the floor (the higher you lift the leg the more difficult the movement). Drop your foot down to the floor and lightly touch the toe on the ground then lift it again. Repeat for 30 seconds then switch sides.

Standing Single Leg Back Beats

Stand with your feet hip distance apart with your desk or a chair that will not move directly to your left. Place your left hand on your desk or chair to steady yourself then shift all your weight onto your left foot, keeping your torso erect and spine tall. Lift your right leg backwards as you point the toe. Lift your foot anywhere from 1 to 12 inches off the floor (the higher you lift the leg the more difficult the movement). Drop your foot down to the floor and lightly touch the toe on the ground then lift it again. Repeat for 30 seconds then switch sides.

Two Full Moons

Stand with your feet slightly wider than hip distance apart. Bend your knees slightly (the deeper you bend your knees the more challenging this exercise becomes). Now tuck your tailbone under your spine, lengthening the lower back. Let your arms dangle at your sides. Roll your shoulders gently open and relax the chest. Allow your head to float off your shoulders. Inhale deeply through your nose as you slowly raise your arms in front of you, palms facing down towards the ground, muscles relaxed and soft until your arms are up over your head. Swing both arms out to your sides as you exhale and lower your arms back down to your sides. Repeat 5 times.

Sweet and Sour (Balance Focused)

Sumo Step

Stand with legs twice hip width apart. Drop the buttocks down six to 10 inches bringing you into a wide legged squat position (the deeper the squat the more challenging this becomes). Shift your weight over to your right foot and slowly lift your left foot off the ground 1 to 8 inches. Hold for a count of 5 then slowly lower the left foot back to the ground. Repeat on the opposite side. Repeat the entire exercise 5 times.

Standing Single Leg Circles

Stand with your feet at hip distance apart with your desk or a chair that will not move directly to your left. Place your left hand on your desk or chair to steady yourself then shift all your weight onto your left foot, keeping your torso erect and spine tall. Lift your right leg out to the side pointing your toe at the floor (your foot should be about six inches off the floor). Make a circle with your foot about the size of a volleyball for 15 seconds. Switch sides.

Pec (pectoral) Stretch

From a standing position bring both hands together behind your back and interlace the fingers. Press your chest out as you lift the joined hands upward, towards the backs of your shoulders. Hold for 30 seconds.

Hip Swivels

Stand with your feet hip distance apart. Place your hands on your hips and slowly start to roll your hips in a circle. With each swivel of your hips make the circles a little bigger. After 30 seconds, switch directions.

Raising your Internal Temperature

Stand with your feet at hip distance apart. Begin to march in place very slowly raising your right leg to a slow count of 3 then lowering it to a slow count of 3 then do the same with the left foot. Continue alternating for 10 to 20 seconds.

Bird on a Perch (Balance Focused)

Raising your Internal Temperature

Stand with your feet at hip distance apart. Begin to march in place very slowly raising your right leg to a slow count of 3 then lowering it to a slow count of 3 then do the same with the left foot. Continue alternating for 30 seconds.

Empty Step

Stand with your feet at hip distance apart. Shift all of your weight onto your left foot and slowly lift your right foot off the ground. Bring your knee up slowly until it is even with your hip. Extend your right foot and bend the left knee touching the toe of the right foot on the floor about 12 inches in front of you, putting no weight on your right foot (as if you were testing the temperature of the water in a lake you were thinking of swimming in). Hold for 30 seconds. Lift your knee back up to hip level then return to your starting position. Switch legs.

Dog Wags His Tail (Modified)

From Wu Chi Stance, bring your hands down to the fronts of your thighs and rest them there. Bend your knees a little deeper, but be sure to keep the tailbone tucked under the spine, lower back long. Now slowly shift all of your weight over to your right foot and pause there for a moment (for more of a challenge, lift your left heel off the ground with only the toe touching).Then with both feet firmly on the ground again shift your weight over to your left foot and pause for a moment (you can lift the right heel if you wish). Go back and forth between the two feet 3 or 4 times.

Turning the Head

Begin in a standing position with arms hanging at your sides and the palms of your hands facing your body. *Very slowly* turn your head to the right and look over your right shoulder as you rotate the palms of your hands out so that they point out and away from your body. *Very slowly* turn your head back so that you are looking forward again as you rotate your palms back so that they face your body again. *Very slowly* turn your head to the left and look over your left shoulder as you rotate your palms out so that they point out and away from your body. *Very slowly* turn your head back so that you are looking forward again as you rotate your palms back so that they face your body again.

Solar Flare (Energizing Focused)

Bellows Breath

The Bellows Breath is adapted from a yogic breathing technique. Its aim is to raise vital energy and increase alertness.

- Inhale and exhale rapidly through your nose, keeping your mouth closed but relaxed. Your breaths in and out should be equal in duration, but as short as possible. This is a noisy breathing exercise.
- Try for 3 in-and-out breath cycles per second. This produces a quick movement of the diaphragm,

suggesting a bellows. Breathe normally after each cycle.

Raising your Internal Temperature

Stand with your feet at hip distance apart. Begin to march in place very slowly raising your right leg to a slow count of 3 then lowering it to a slow count of 3 then do the same with the left foot. Continue alternating for 10 to 20 seconds.

Two Full Moons

Stand with your feet slightly wider than hip distance apart. Bend your knees slightly (the deeper you bend your knees the more challenging this exercise becomes). Now tuck your tailbone under your spine, lengthening the lower back. Let your arms dangle at your sides. Roll your shoulders gently open and relax the chest. Allow your head to float off your shoulders. Inhale deeply through your nose as you slowly raise your arms in front of you, palms facing down towards the ground, muscles relaxed and soft until your arms are up over your head. Swing both arms out to your sides as you exhale and lower your arms back down to your sides. Repeat for 30 seconds.

Awakening the Chi

From a standing position with feet at hip distance apart bend your knees slightly. Inhale deeply through your nose then slowly exhale out through your mouth. Continue to breathe like this the entire time you do the rest of the movements. Take your hands and begin to slap the fronts of your thighs vigorously. You should feel the area being slapped begin to feel tingly; if it hurts you're slapping too hard. Move to the backs of your thighs, then up to the buttocks. Move up the body slapping the fronts of your hips, belly, chest, shoulders, arms and finally the face. Make the entirety of this movement last for about 1 minute.

Dancing Child (Energizing Focused)

Hip Swivels

Stand with your feet hip distance apart. Place your hands on your hips and slowly start to roll your hips in a circle. With each swivel of your hips make the circles a little bigger. After 30 seconds, switch directions.

Swimming on Land

Stand with your feet slightly wider than hip distance apart. Bend your knees slightly (the deeper you bend your knees the more challenging this exercise becomes). Now tuck your tailbone under your spine, lengthening the lower back. Bring your hands up in front of your chest, elbows pointing outward. Start to move your hands as if you were doing the breast stroke (a wide circular motion at chest height). Inhale deeply through your nose and exhale slowly through your mouth as you continue to "swim" with your arms. Do this for 20 breaths.

Awakening the Chi

From a standing position with your feet hip distance apart, bend your knees slightly. Inhale deeply through your nose then slowly exhale out through your mouth. Continue to breathe like this the entire time you do the rest of the movements. Take your hands and begin to slap the fronts of your thighs vigorously. You should feel the area being slapped begin to feel tingly; if it hurts, you're slapping too hard. Move to the backs of the thighs, then up to the buttocks. Move up the body slapping the fronts of the hips, belly, chest, shoulders, arms and finally the face. Make the entirety of this movement last for about 1 minute.

Opening the Door

Stand with your feet slightly wider than hip distance apart. Bend your knees slightly (the deeper you bend your knees the more challenging this movement becomes). Now tuck your tailbone under your spine, lengthening the lower back. Let your arms dangle at your sides. Roll your shoulders gently open and relax the chest. Allow your head to float off your shoulders. Inhale deeply through your nose as you slowly raise your arms in front of you, palms facing down towards the ground, muscles relaxed and soft until your arms reach shoulder height. Raise your palms so that they face forward and exhale through your mouth as you slowly lower your arms back down to their original position. Repeat 20 times.

Nuclear Reactor (Energizing Focused)

Alternate Nostril Breathing

Alternate nostril breathing creates optimum function of both sides of the brain, improves mood, strengthens the lungs and energizes the body.

- Close off the right nostril with your right thumb then inhale through the left nostril to a three-count
- Hold your breath for an eight-count
- Release your thumb from your right nostril and exhale through the right nostril for a count of 6 as you close off the left nostril with your left thumb.
- Now inhale through your right nostril for a three-count and repeat this on both sides for 1 to 3 minutes.

Shake Illness from the Body

Begin in a standing position, feet hip distance apart, arms hanging at the sides of the body. Lift up onto your toes as high as you can and pause. Drop down heavily on the soles of your feet and shake the body and arms vigorously (if this brings you pain simply drop down gentl0y, minimizing the bang at the bottom). Repeat 3 to 4 times.

Awakening the Chi

From a standing position with your feet hip distance apart, bend your knees slightly. Inhale deeply through your nose then slowly exhale out through your mouth. Continue to breathe like this the entire time you do the rest of the movements. Take your hands and begin to slap the fronts of your thighs vigorously. You should feel the area being slapped begin to feel tingly; if it hurts, you're slapping too hard. Move to the backs of the thighs, then up to the buttocks. Move up the body slapping the fronts of the hips, belly, chest, shoulders, arms and finally the face. Make the entirety of this movement last for about 1 minute.

Lifting the Sky

Bring your hands up in front of your hips, palms facing up as if you were supporting a large belly in front of you. Slowly pull your palms up towards your chin, keeping your hands a few inches away from the front of your body. When your hands reach your chest rotate the palms down, forward and up until your palms face the sky, and press upward until your arms are extended overhead as if lifting the sky. When your arms are fully extended overhead allow them to swing outward in a wide arc to your sides coming slowly back to the original position.

Happy Puppy (Energizing Focused)

Looking Back at the Moon

Stand with your feet slightly wider than hip distance apart facing forward. Place both hands on your hips and slowly twist at the waist as you turn your entire upper body to the left. Be sure to keep your feet firmly planted on the floor. Turn your head to the left as if looking behind you and hold for 5 seconds. Switch sides.

Opening the Door

Stand with your feet slightly wider than hip distance apart. Bend your knees slightly (the deeper you bend your knees the more challenging this movement becomes). Now tuck your tailbone under your spine, lengthening the lower back. Let your arms dangle at your sides. Roll your shoulders gently open and relax the chest. Allow your head to float off your shoulders. Inhale deeply through your nose as you slowly raise your arms in front of you, palms facing down towards the ground, muscles relaxed and soft until your arms reach shoulder height. Raise your palms so that they face forward and exhale through your mouth as you slowly lower your arms back down to their original position. Repeat 20 times.

Pulling the Bow

Stand with your feet slightly wider than hip distance apart. Swing your elbows outward as you bring your hands up to your chest, palms facing the body. Ball your hands into fists (tops of the fists should be facing one another). The next movement is like an archer pulling his bow: keeping the left hand where it is, slowly extend your right arm out to the right side at shoulder height as if ready to the shoot the arrow. Hold for a moment feeling the tension between the bow and the string. Slowly bring your right hand back to your chest. Keep the right hand were it is and slowly extend your left arm out to the left side at shoulder height as if ready to shoot the arrow. Hold for a moment feeling the tension between the bow and the string. Slowly bring the left hand back to your chest.

Chair-Supported Downward Facing Dog

Rise from your seated position and walk behind your chair. Secure the chair so that it will not move or roll away. Facing the back of the chair, grab the top of the chair back and then take a step or two backwards away from the chair until your arms are fully extended. Hinge at the hips and lean forward bringing the torso parallel to the floor beneath you. You should feel a gentle stretch in the low back and hamstring muscles. Hold for 30 seconds.

Five Minute Activity Segments

Blue Moon Rising (Flexibility Focused)

Lifting the Sky

Bring your hands up in front of your hips, palms facing up as if you were supporting a large belly in front of you. Slowly pull your palms up towards your chin, keeping your hands a few inches away from the front of your body. When your hands reach your chest rotate the palms down, forward and up until your palms face the sky, and press upward until your arms are extended overhead as if lifting the sky. When your arms are fully extended overhead allow them to swing outward in a wide arc to your sides coming slowly back to the original position. Repeat 5 times.

Wide Leg Turnout Squat

Stand with your arms folded at your chest. Spread your legs so they are twice hip distance apart with toes pointed outward at a 45-degree angle from the mid-line of the body. Bend your knees as you drop your buttocks down towards the floor as if you were going to sit in a chair but be sure to keep your torso as upright as possible. Then return to the starting position. Repeat for 1 minute.

Modified Hanging Pose

Begin in a standing position with feet hip distance apart. Bend both knees slightly, then lean forward and slowly lower your head as you begin to reach down toward your mid-thighs or knees depending on what feels comfortable for you. Support the upper body with your hands, and allow the spine to lengthen toward the floor as much as feels comfortable. Hold this pose for 1 minute while taking long, slow, deep breaths.

Looking Back at the Moon

Stand with your feet slightly wider than hip distance apart facing forward. Place both hands on your hips and slowly twist at the waist as you turn your entire upper body to the left. Be sure to keep your feet firmly planted on the floor. Turn your head to the left as if looking behind you and hold for 30 seconds. Switch sides.

Bending to the Sides

Stand with your feet slightly wider than hip distance apart. Place your right hand on your right hip. Bring your left hand up over your head as you gently lean to the right, pressing your left hip out to the left. Reach with your left hand over your head until you feel a gentle stretch all along your left side. Hold for 30 seconds then switch sides.

Falcon Soars (Flexibility Focused)

Two Full Moons

Stand with your feet slightly wider than hip distance apart. Bend your knees slightly (the deeper you bend your knees the more challenging this exercise becomes). Now tuck your tailbone under your spine, lengthening the lower back. Let your arms dangle at your sides. Roll your shoulders gently open and relax the chest. Allow your head to float off your shoulders. Inhale deeply through your nose as you slowly raise your arms in front of you, palms facing down towards the ground, muscles relaxed and soft until your arms are up over your head. Swing both arms out to your sides as you exhale and lower your arms back down to your sides. Repeat for 1 minute.

Half Eagle

You can do this one from either the standing or seated position. Bring your left arm directly out in front of you at chest level, bend the elbow and point your forearm and hand up towards the sky. Take your right arm and cross the right bicep under your left elbow as you reach with your right hand up and around your left forearm grabbing the inside of the left wrist. Hold for 30 seconds then switch sides.

Triceps Stretch

You can do this one from either the standing or seated position. Reach up towards the ceiling with your right arm then drop your right hand down behind your head, pointing your right elbow up towards the ceiling. Reach up to your right elbow with your left hand and gently pull the elbow towards the midline of your body until you feel a gentle stretch in the back of your right tricep. Hold for 30 seconds then switch arms.

Quad & Hip Flexor Stretch

Stand and hold onto a chair or your desk with your left hand. Bend your right knee bringing your right heel up towards your buttocks. Reach down and grab your right ankle. Pull your knee cap down towards the floor and press your right hip gently forward. Hold for 30 seconds. Switch sides.

Pec (pectoral) Stretch

From a standing position bring both hands together behind your back and interlace the fingers. Press your chest out as you lift the joined hands upward, towards the backs of your shoulders. Hold for 1 minute.

Mountain Brook (Flexibility Focused)

Neck Rolls

Stand with your feet hip distance apart, arms hanging down to your sides. Gently roll your head in small circles and then slowly make each circle a little bigger. After 30 seconds, reverse the direction of your circles.

Pushing the Wall

Stand facing a clear wall. Rest both hands on the wall at chest height. Bend your elbows slightly. Step back as far as you can with your right foot then press into the wall firmly. Continue to press into the wall for 30 seconds. Switch legs and repeat.

Calf Stretch

From a standing position turn and face your desk or wall. Place the palms of your hands on the desk or wall and bend your left knee slightly as you take your right foot and step back. Press your heel down towards the ground and lean gently forward. You should feel a gentle stretch at the back of your lower right leg. Hold for 30 seconds then switch legs.

Hamstring Stretch

From a standing position step forward with your right foot approximately 2 feet keeping your right knee straight but not locked. Hinge at the hips, leaning forward until you feel a gentle stretch in the back of the right thigh. Hold for 30 seconds and switch legs.

Quad & Hip Flexor Stretch

Stand and hold onto a chair or your desk with your left hand. Bend your right knee bringing your right heel up towards your buttocks. Reach down and grab your right ankle. Pull your knee cap down towards the floor and press your right hip gently forward. Hold for 30 seconds. Switch sides.

The Languid Eel (Flexibility Focused)

Hip Swivels

Stand with your feet hip distance apart. Place your hands on your hips and slowly start to roll your hips in a circle. With each swivel of your hips make the circles a little bigger. After 30 seconds, switch directions.

Bending Backwards

Stand with your feet slightly wider than hip distance apart. Now tuck your tailbone under your spine, lengthening the lower back. Place both hands behind you at the small of your back and gently lean backwards. As you begin to lean back, bend your knees slightly and press your hips forward. Allow your chest to rise upward as you look up at the ceiling. Hold for 10 seconds and return to the starting position. Repeat 6 times.

Bending to the sides

Stand with your feet slightly wider than hip distance apart. Place your right hand on your right hip. Bring your left hand up over your head as you gently lean to the right, pressing your left hip out to the left. Reach with your left hand over your head until you feel a gentle stretch all along your left side. Hold for 30 seconds then switch sides.

Ankle Circles

Stand with your feet hip distance apart. Shift all of your weight onto your left foot and slowly lift your right foot off the ground. Balance there on your left foot for a breath or two then slowly roll the right foot in a circle for 15 seconds. Slowly bring the right foot back down to the ground and repeat with the left foot.

Modified Hanging Pose

Begin in a standing position with feet hip distance apart. Bend both knees slightly, then lean forward and slowly lower your head as you begin to reach down toward your mid-thighs or knees depending on what feels comfortable for you. Support the upper body with your hands, and allow the spine to lengthen toward the floor as much as feels comfortable. Hold this pose for 1 minute while taking long, slow, deep breaths.

War Hammer (Strength Focused)

Punch with Eye Glaring

Stand with your feet slightly wider than hip distance apart. Making sure that your tailbone is tucked under, bring your hands up so that your hands and wrists are in line with your elbows, palms facing up, elbows pressed against your ribcage. Ball your fists and draw the elbows back until your wrists are pressed against your ribcage. Give me your best Kung Fu glare as you punch with your right hand, slowly rotating the hand so that the palm faces the ground, moving slowly like you were punching in mud. Pull your hand back and repeat with the left hand. Continue for 1 minute.

Lateral Raises

Stand with your feet slightly wider than hip distance apart. Drop your arms down to your sides. Keeping your arms long and straight raise them until they reach shoulder height then lower them back to your sides. Repeat for 1 minute.

Pushing the Wall

Stand facing a clear wall. Rest both hands on the wall at chest height. Bend your elbows slightly. Step back as far as you can with your right foot then press into the wall firmly. Continue to press into the wall for 30 seconds. Switch legs and repeat.

Swimming on Land

Stand with your feet slightly wider than hip distance apart. Bend your knees slightly (the deeper you bend your knees the more challenging this exercise becomes). Now tuck your tailbone under your spine, lengthening the lower back. Bring your hands up in front of your chest, elbows pointing outward. Start to move your hands as if you were doing the breast stroke (a wide circular motion at chest height). Inhale deeply through your nose and exhale slowly through your mouth as you continue to "swim" with your arms. Do this for 20 breaths.

Wide Leg Turnout Squat

Stand with your arms folded at your chest. Spread your legs so they are twice hip distance apart with toes pointed outward at a 45-degree angle from the mid-line of the body. Bend your knees as you drop your buttocks down towards the floor as if you were going to sit in a chair but be sure to keep your torso as upright as possible. Then return to the starting position. Repeat for 1 minute.

Lightning Strikes (Strength Focused)

Pushing the Wall

Stand facing a clear wall. Rest both hands on the wall at chest height. Bend your elbows slightly. Step back as far as you can with your right foot then press into the wall firmly. Continue to press into the wall for 30 seconds. Switch legs and repeat.

Tree Pose (modified)

Stand with your feet hip distance apart. Shift your weight onto your left foot and bring your right foot off the ground. Place the sole of your right foot against the calf of your left leg. Bring the palms of your hands together in prayer position in the middle of your chest then forcefully push them together. Hold for 30 seconds then switch legs.

Lunge

Stand with your feet slightly wider than hip distance apart. Place both hands on your hips. Step forward with your right foot approximately 18 to 24 inches. Bend your left knee and slowly kneel until the left knee touches or almost touches the floor. Be sure to keep the torso upright and the spine long. Keeping your feet where they are, slowly stand, then lower the left knee back to the floor. Repeat for 30 seconds then switch sides.

Quad & Hip Flexor Stretch

Stand and hold onto a chair or your desk with your left hand. Bend your right knee bringing your right heel up towards your buttocks. Reach down and grab your right ankle. Pull your knee cap down towards the floor and press your right hip gently forward. Hold for 30 seconds. Switch sides.

Side-Step Lunge

Begin in a standing position with feet hip distance apart. Step with the right foot to the right about 12 inches. Keep the left knee straight and bend the right knee, leaning out towards your right foot until you feel a gentle stretch on the inside of your left leg. Hold for 30 seconds then switch sides.

Scales (Balance Focused)

Tree Pose (modified)

Stand with your feet hip distance apart. Shift your weight onto your left foot and bring your right foot off the ground. Place the sole of your right foot against the calf of your left leg. Bring the palms of your hands together in prayer position in the middle of your chest then forcefully push them together. Hold for 30 seconds then switch legs.

Standing Single Leg Circles

Stand with your feet at hip distance apart with your desk or a chair that will not move directly to your left. Place your left hand on your desk or chair to steady yourself then shift all your weight onto your left foot, keeping your torso erect and spine tall. Lift your right leg out to the side pointing your toe at the floor (your foot should be about six inches off the floor). Make a circle about the size of a volleyball with your foot for 30 seconds. Switch sides.

Lifting the Knee

Stand with your feet hip distance apart. Shift all your weight onto your left foot and slowly lift your right foot off the ground. Bring your knee up slowly until it is even with your hip (thigh should be parallel to the floor), hold it there for 30 seconds, then slowly lower it back down to the floor. Switch legs.

Wu Chi Stance

Stand with your feet slightly wider than hip distance apart. Bend your knees slightly (the deeper you bend your knees the more challenging this exercise becomes). Now tuck your tailbone under the spine, lengthening the lower back. Let your arms dangle at your sides. Roll your shoulders gently open and relax the chest. Allow your head to float off your shoulders. Hold for 1 minute.

Shoulder Rolls

Stand with your feet hip distance apart, arms hanging down to your sides. Gently roll the shoulders forward, down and back making as big a circle with the shoulders as you comfortably can. After 30 seconds, reverse the direction of your circles.

The Unicycle (Balance Focused)

Ankle Circles

Stand with your feet hip distance apart. Shift all of your weight onto your left foot and slowly lift your right foot off the ground. Balance there on your left foot for a breath or two then slowly roll the right foot in a circle for 30 seconds. Slowly bring the right foot back down to the ground and repeat with the left foot.

Standing Single Leg Circles

Stand with your feet at hip distance apart with your desk or a chair that will not move directly to your left. Place your left hand on your desk or chair to steady yourself then shift all your weight onto your left foot, keeping your torso erect and spine tall. Lift your right leg out to the side pointing your toe at the floor (your foot should be about six inches off the floor). Make a circle with your foot about the size of a volleyball for 30 seconds. Switch sides.

Chair Dips

Sit on an immovable chair or desk. Place your hands on either side of your hips with your palms flat on the desk or the seat of the chair, fingers pointed forward. With your feet on the floor, walk your feet as far away from you as you can, sliding your buttocks off the edge of the chair or desk. After your buttocks has cleared the edge of the chair or desk and is hovering off the ground, your body supported by your arms and feet, keep the knees bent and aligned over the ankles. If you would like a little more of a challenge you can extend your legs and balance on your heels. Keeping the core engaged and the butt lifted, lower your body down towards the ground, then press back up to original starting position. Repeat for 30 seconds. Rest and repeat for 30 seconds more.

Looking back at the moon

Stand with your feet slightly wider than hip distance apart facing forward. Place both hands on your hips and slowly twist at the waist as you turn your entire upper body to the left. Be sure to keep your feet firmly planted on the floor. Turn your head to the left as if looking behind you and hold for 30 seconds. Switch sides.

Standing Single Leg Back Beats

Stand with your feet hip distance apart with your desk or a chair that will not move directly to your left. Place your left hand on your desk or chair to steady yourself then shift all your weight onto your left foot, keeping your torso erect and spine tall. Lift your right leg backwards as you point the toe. Lift your foot anywhere from 1 to 12 inches off the floor (the higher you lift the leg the more difficult the movement). Drop your foot down to the floor and lightly touch the toe on the ground then lift it again. Repeat for 30 seconds then switch sides.

Erupting Volcano (Energizing Focused)

Alternate Nostril Breathing

Alternate nostril breathing creates optimum function of both sides of the brain, improves mood, strengthens the lungs and energizes the body.

- Close off the right nostril with your right thumb then inhale through the left nostril to a three-count
- Hold your breath for an eight-count
- Release your thumb from your right nostril and exhale through the right nostril for a count of 6 as you close off the left nostril with your left thumb.
- Now inhale through your right nostril for a three-count and repeat this on both sides for 1 to 3 minutes.

Wide Leg Turnout Squat

Stand with your arms folded at your chest. Spread your legs so they are twice hip distance apart with toes pointed outward at a 45-degree angle from the mid-line of the body. Bend your knees as you drop your buttocks down towards the floor as if you were going to sit in a chair but be sure to keep your torso as upright as possible. Then return to the starting position. Repeat for 1 minute.

Awakening the Chi

From a standing position with your feet hip distance apart, bend your knees slightly. Inhale deeply through your nose then slowly exhale out through your mouth. Continue to breathe like this the entire time you do the rest of the movements. Take your hands and begin to slap the fronts of your thighs vigorously. You should feel the area being slapped begin to feel tingly; if it hurts, you're slapping too hard. Move to the backs of the thighs, then up to the buttocks. Move up the body slapping the fronts of the hips, belly, chest, shoulders, arms and finally the face. Make the entirety of this movement last for about 1 minute.

Two Full Moons

Stand with your feet slightly wider than hip distance apart. Bend your knees slightly (the deeper you bend your knees the more challenging this exercise becomes). Now tuck your tailbone under your spine, lengthening the lower back. Let your arms dangle at your sides. Roll your shoulders gently open and relax the chest. Allow your head to float off your shoulders. Inhale deeply through your nose as you slowly raise your arms in front of you, palms facing down towards the ground, muscles relaxed and soft until your arms are up over your head. Swing both arms out to your sides as you exhale and lower your arms back down to your sides. Repeat 10 times.

Lifting the Sky

Bring your hands up in front of your hips, palms facing up as if you were supporting a large belly in front of you. Slowly pull your palms up towards your chin, keeping your hands a few inches away from the front of your body. When your hands reach your chest rotate the palms down, forward and up until your palms face the sky, and press upward until your arms are extended overhead as if lifting the sky. When your arms are fully extended overhead allow them to swing outward in a wide arc to your sides coming slowly back to the original position. Repeat for 1 minute.

Forceful Geyser (Energizing Focused)

Bellows Breath

The Bellows Breath is adapted from a yogic breathing technique. Its aim is to raise vital energy and increase alertness.

- Inhale and exhale rapidly through your nose, keeping your mouth closed but relaxed. Your breaths in and out should be equal in duration, but as short as possible. This is a noisy breathing exercise.

- Try for 3 in-and-out breath cycles per second. This produces a quick movement of the diaphragm, suggesting a bellows. Breathe normally after each cycle.

Swimming on Land

Stand with your feet slightly wider than hip distance apart. Bend your knees slightly (the deeper you bend your knees the more challenging this exercise becomes). Now tuck your tailbone under your spine, lengthening the lower back. Bring your hands up in front of your chest, elbows pointing outward. Start to move your hands as if you were doing the breast stroke (a wide circular motion at chest height). Inhale deeply through your nose and exhale slowly through your mouth as you continue to "swim" with your arms. Do this for 1 minute.

Pushing the Wall

Stand facing a clear wall. Rest both hands on the wall at chest height. Bend your elbows slightly. Step back as far as you can with your right foot then press into the wall firmly. Continue to press into the wall for 30 seconds. Switch legs and repeat.

Two Full Moons

Stand with your feet slightly wider than hip distance apart. Bend your knees slightly (the deeper you bend your knees the more challenging this exercise becomes). Now tuck your tailbone under your spine, lengthening the lower back. Let your arms dangle at your sides. Roll your shoulders gently open and relax the chest. Allow your head to float off your shoulders. Inhale deeply through your nose as you slowly raise your arms in front of you, palms facing down towards the ground, muscles relaxed and soft until your arms are up over your head. Swing both arms out to your sides as you exhale and lower your arms back down to your sides. Repeat 10 times.

Lateral Raises

Stand with your feet slightly wider than hip distance apart. Drop your arms down to your sides. Keeping your arms long and straight raise them until they reach shoulder height then lower them back to your sides. Repeat for 1 minute.

Sample 1 Week Program

I have created a one-week sample program to give you an idea of how you can put together your own program from the movement section of this book. I have also added some suggestions for adding exercise to your schedule. As I've said several times in this book, regular exercise is important to your overall health and is especially helpful in keeping your weight at a healthy level. All of the times indicated are *minimum suggestions,* so please feel free to do more than the samples. Although the sample is based on an eight-hour work day with a one-hour lunch break, I am aware that your work day may be very different than this. However, the movements in the program are specifically designed so that you can adjust them according to your own schedule. Also note that I have put the exercise at the end of the day because I happen to be an evening person. If you prefer the mornings, you can move the exercise to before work. The main thing is to create a schedule that works for you. The easier this is, the more likely you are to do it regularly and that is the key to making this truly helpful to your overall wellbeing.

While we are on the subject, I would like to talk a little about the reputation of that word, "exercise." I know that for many people "exercise" is a dirty word, and many people simply despise exercising. They don't like the way it feels, they don't like getting sweaty and they don't like doing things they feel haven't brought them a great deal of success in the past. For some, exercise brings up bad memories of mean

P.E. teachers and being picked last for teams in gym class. If you are one of those people, take heart; you don't have to "exercise" to be healthy, but you do have to be active and there is a big difference. So if slinging around a bunch of heavy dumbbells, doing a boot camp class or trying to keep up with that maniac on the P90X video isn't your idea of a good time, that's okay. There are other things you can do to be active that you may find more enjoyable—I'll even go as far as to say fun— that will keep you fit and healthy.

First on that list is walking. Like I stated in the very first chapter of this book, walking is exactly what our bodies were created to do. You don't need any special equipment to walk (good shoes are a plus, but people all over the globe walk barefoot all the time). You don't need a membership in a gym or a personal trainer to tell you how to do it (though you can use those things to walk if you want to). Personally, my very favorite thing in the world to do is to find a secluded trail and go walking in the countryside, just like our ancestors did. It feels great, I see a bunch of beautiful scenery and it does wonders for my body, mind and spirit. Some other great options are bicycling, kayaking, rock climbing, surfing, boogie boarding, stand-up paddling, racquetball, yoga, Pilates, tai chi or dancing, just to name a few... The great news is that today there are more ways than ever to start doing any one of these activities. I have talked to many people who have fallen in love with the new dance games offered by the Wii, Xbox and PlayStation game makers. These games allow you to dance in the privacy of your home to the hottest dance music while getting one heck of a work out. Extra bonus: they basically teach you the steps to the latest dances being done at the clubs and on music videos (at least that's what I've been told. I haven't been to a club since dinosaurs ruled the Earth). The point here is that being active can actually be a lot of fun so explore your options and then get yourself moving with something you really enjoy doing.

Monday

9:45am	Minute Flexibility	Curling Serpent
10:45am	1 Minute Strength	Ancient Mountain
11:45am	3 Minute Energizing	Solar Flare
12:45pm	5 Minute Flexibility	Mountain Brook
1:45pm	1 Minute Balance	Yin/Yang
2:45pm	1 Minute Strength	Hunting Tiger
3:45pm	3 Minute Energizing	Dancing Child
4:45pm	1 Minute Balance	The Flamingo
6:00pm	30-60 Minute brisk walk, jog, dance etc.	

Tuesday

9:45am	1 Minute Balance	Ninja on the Roof
10:45am	1 Minute Flexibility	Awakening Cat
11:45am	3 Minute Strength	Tsunami
12:45pm	5 Minute Energizing	Spurting Geyser
1:45pm	1 Minute Balance	Ninja on the Roof
2:45pm	1 Minute Strength	Mother Bear
3:45pm	3 Minute Balance	Bird on a Perch
4:45pm	1 Minute Flexibility	Swaying Palm
6:00pm	30-60 Minute brisk walk, jog, dance etc.	

Wednesday

9:45am	1 Minute Strength	Mighty Wind
10:45am	1 Minute Balance	Ninja on the Roof
11:45am	3 Minute Flexibility	Reeds in the Breeze
12:45pm	5 Minute Energizing	Erupting Volcano
1:45pm	1 Minute Flexibility	Supple Leaf
2:45pm	1 Minute Balance	The Stork
3:45pm	3 Minute Strength	Crashing Thunder
4:45pm	1 Minute Flexibility	Willow Bends in Wind
6:00pm	30-60 Minute brisk walk, jog, dance etc.	

Thursday

9:45am	1 Minute Flexibility	Flowing River
10:45am	1 Minute Energizing	Fast Running Stream
11:45am	3 Minute Strength	The Plough Horse
12:45pm	5 Minute Balance	Scales
1:45pm	1 Minute Flexibility	Awakening Cat
2:45pm	1 Minute Strength	Drunken Elephant
3:45pm	3 Minute Flexibility	Placid Lake
4:45pm	1 Minute Balance	Boulder on a Ridge
6:00pm	30-60 Minute brisk walk, jog, dance etc.	

Friday

9:45am	1 Minute Energizing	Happy Toddler
10:45am	1 Minute Balance	Mountain Goat
11:45am	3 Minute Flexibility	Shifting Sand
12:45pm	5 Minute Strength	War Hammer
1:45pm	1 Minute Energizing	Electric Eel
2:45pm	1 Minute Strength	Brave Warrior
3:45pm	3 Minute Flexibility	Shifting Sand
4:45pm	1 Minute Balance	Ninja on the Roof
6:00pm	30-60 Minute brisk walk, jog, dance etc.	

Saturday

Go out and have some fun. Play a pickup game of basketball, do some gardening, take a yoga class, or play a dance game.

Sunday

Rest

Chapter 6

Over The Top

Are you one of those people who like to do just a little bit more than most other people? Do you need to know the latest research on a subject, need to own the hottest gadgets? Were you were the first in your family, neighborhood, office or town to own the iPod, iPhone or iPad? If so, this chapter is for you. I call this chapter *Over the Top* because what I'm about to talk about is just that. It's over the top. Some people may look at this stuff and say "wow, that's weird!" And in truth they are probably right...for now. But I'm going to go out on a limb here and predict that as we find out more about the dangers and costs of extended periods of sitting, some of the products I discuss in this chapter will become much more commonplace. One of the most telling signs that these products are powerful tools is that virtually every one of the people involved in sedentary studies research uses these products or have created their own variation of the product that they use in their work spaces and homes.

Take Dr. Levine for example. He uses a treadmill desk in his office, where he walks at a steady 1.5 mile per hour pace as he works on the computer, answers phone calls and talks to colleagues. Dr. Hamilton has a stand-up desk in his office, and others report using fitness balls, stationary bike desks and exotic exercise chairs. Some of these products are pricey, but with a little imagination (and maybe some power tools), you can create your own healthy office furniture. I have a friend that simply placed an apple crate on top of her conventional desk to create the perfect height for a stand up desk, and I personally cut a piece of plywood to fit on my home treadmill, strapped it to the arms and stuck my laptop on it to make my own treadmill desk. There is no doubt that if you bring some of this stuff to your work space you are going to be labeled as the office eccentric, but there are some advantages to being the office eccentric; for one, being healthy.

We've seen that standing alone burns 60 calories more each hour than sitting. Over the course of an eight-hour day that is an additional 480 calories burned. Add an additional 40 calories per hour from walking at a pace of 1.5 miles an hour and you're looking at a total 100 calories burned an hour. Add all this up, and it's hard to ignore a count of 800 extra calories burned over just one eight-hour workday, no exercise needed. Not too shabby. So without further ado, let's check out some of these weird, wacky and wonderful products.

Stability Ball

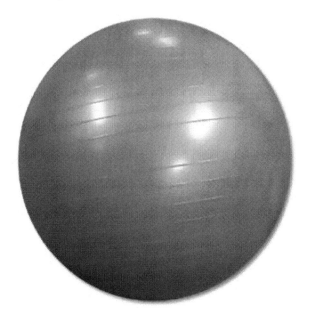

Stability balls have been around forever. Typically, trainers use these to create instability in different exercises, forcing the body to use stabilizer muscles to improve strength and balance. When used as a chair they are really just a half-step up from the traditional chair. You're still in that seated position, which tends to shorten the hip flexors and put strain on the spine. But on a stability ball, you are forced to activate your postural muscles to keep the ball from rolling away. The thigh muscles are also much more active on the ball than on a traditional chair, and for people who are fidgety like me, the ball offers unlimited opportunities to move around. The major downside to the stability ball is that it's super easy to fall off of, which can be a bit embarrassing at the office.

Stand-Up Desk

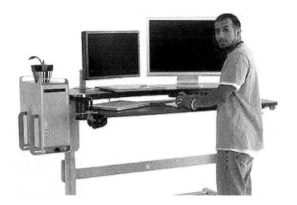

Stand-up desks are desks that are taller than traditional desks and therefore meant to be stood at. These are not new; In fact, author Ernest Hemingway was said to use a stand-up desk, as was Secretary of Defense Donald Rumsfeld. Standing desks take a little getting used to, but most people rave about their standing desks after the adjustment period. Mostly you hear about weight loss, disappearing back pain and increasing energy levels. The major drawback to these desks is the price. Lots of companies make them, including IKEA, but they will set you back between $1,200 and $2,500, and they have to be somewhat customized. I am sure you can imagine that a desk that will accommodate a person who is 4'9" isn't going to be very comfortable for a person who is 6' 5". I have seen several money-saving designs, such as putting desks up on boxes, and placing monitors and keyboards on flat boards resting on full cases of canned soft drinks. Don't be afraid to think outside the box; this is one of those cases where a little imagination can get you a healthier workspace for very little money.

Stationary Bike Desk

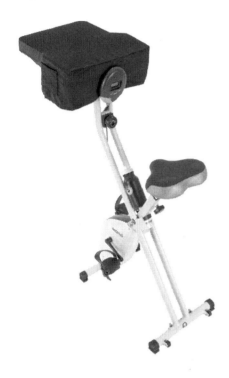

The stationary bike desk concept was popular among several of the researchers mentioned in this book. Again, you're still in that seated position but muscle activation in the postural muscles and the legs is pretty heavy with this concept, and the calorie burn is significant. It also has the advantage of being really safe, even for those with very little body awareness (that's a polite term for people like my wife, which is to say *a little klutzy*). They are safe because falling off the bike is far less likely to occur if you get distracted by a call or email and forget to move your feet. You can get more information on this bike desk at *www.fitdesk.net*. At the time of publication the Fitdesk will cost you about $229.99 plus tax, shipping and handling. One researcher saved some money by putting together a simple peddle machine under his desk that he peddled throughout the day.

Treadmill Desks

A treadmill desk is the Rolls Royce of healthy office furniture from a calorie-burning and postural-muscle-engaging standpoint—it's also the most expensive option. These desks incorporate exactly what our body was created to do with the ease of use that a traditional desk supplies. Heck, several models even actually incorporate cup holders in the design! The walking pace can be controlled so that you don't feel overwhelmed or get sweaty. The work space can be raised or lowered for ultimate comfort and the daily calorie burn is huge. The learning curve for most people is about 3 hours, but after that, the term I've heard most often used to describe the experience is "addictive." The secret seems to be to find the perfect speed for you. Too slow and you can't find a rhythm. Too fast and you'll feel like you're going to fall off while you do your basic daily tasks. But once you find your sweet spot, it's like nirvana. In addition to the physical benefits, most researchers also talked about better brain function and claimed they felt more alert and focused throughout the day. Personally, I know that I think more clearly and get more done when I'm walking. In fact, I tend to do my best work while on the move, so the walking desk fits me to a tee. If you're interested in walking and working at the same time you have a couple of different options. One, if you don't currently have a treadmill, one option is to buy a treadmill that has a desk integrated or attached to it, like the Lifespan TR1200 treadmill desk pictured below:

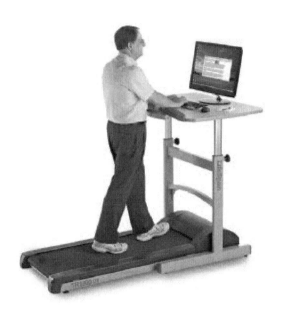

www.lifespanfitness.com/treadmill-desk.asp

If you plan to use this equipment day in and day out at low speeds, well, traditional treadmills aren't really designed for that and may not last very long. In the long haul, a complete system like this one may be a better purchase.

However, if you already own a treadmill you can always just buy a desk for it, like the TrekDesk (pictured below). This is a product that is specifically designed to simply fit over the treadmill you already own.

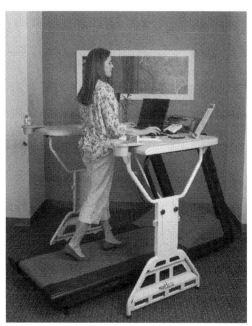

www.trekdesk.com

As I mentioned earlier, I accomplished this myself with some power tools and a little elbow grease (though in all fairness, mine is pretty shoddy looking and doesn't have anywhere near the work surface area or cool cup holders).

These are just a few of the products on the market that will help you work in a healthier way. A simple Google search will yield many additional options depending on your focus and interest. There are many "exercise chairs" that incorporate bands and weights and have other bells and whistles. But rather than being seduced by the marketing hype of these chairs, try to keep in mind that getting OUT of the chair is much better than just exercising in a seated position.

Chapter 7

Conclusion

Writing this book has opened my eyes to an entirely new way of thinking about health and wellness. I've always known that being a couch potato isn't a stop on the path to wellness and that living a sedentary lifestyle increases the chance of developing a life-threatening disease. This new research is redefining what constitutes an active lifestyle. When you look at the biology of sitting and the chemical and hormonal processes that take place in our bodies when we sit, we are forced to look at sitting in a new light. Our bodies were designed to be active all day long. Our hunter gatherer ancestors walked long distances in search of food and patrolling their territory while carrying their few belongings with them wherever they roamed. Later our farmer ancestors tilled their fields, weeded their gardens and tended their animals for food and for trade. They did these things constantly over the course of the day because their lives depended on it; keeping food on the table required it.

Today our lives and livelihoods no longer require us to be as active, but ignoring hundreds of thousands of years of evolution has brought serious consequences. Look around and you will see the price we're paying. If you yourself are not suffering from obesity, heart disease, diabetes or cancer or in the process of developing one of them, then you surely know someone who is. These lifestyle diseases eat away at personal health and wellbeing as well as our social and economic health and wellbeing. These conditions cost countless lives and billions of dollars each year. Let me be clear: I am not asserting that getting out of your chair regularly will completely eliminate the risk of developing a serious disease. Getting up and moving often can, however, substantially decrease those risks.

In this book I have given you simple yet powerful ways to make a change in your sitting patterns. The movements are easy to do, engage the all-important postural muscles and encourage better blood flow throughout the body. The movements can be done individually or put together to create a short break that both refreshes the mind and body as well as works on strength, balance and flexibility. The latest research suggests that doing the movements frequently is more important than doing them for a long duration; doing three one-minute movements over the course of an hour seems to be more effective than doing one three minute movement segment in an hour.

I believe that simplicity is the key to success when it comes to making lasting changes in your life; these movements are definitely simple. For those looking for something a little more exotic there are the ball chairs, standing desks, walking desks and even bike desks. No matter what you chose to do, doing something is the key, and then, *do it often* until it just becomes what you do.

This is all very new research and in the coming years we will learn more about frequency of movement and what types of movements or exercises will maximize your effort and time. In the meantime just getting up and out of the seated position and moving around and balancing and stretching on a regular basis will get you headed in the right direction. Some people will say that this research is too preliminary, that there isn't enough data to reach any solid conclusions about sitting. Maybe they're right. But tell me this; what's the downside to being more active? How is doing these movements going to be detrimental to your health? You can sit around and wait for more research to come in as your health slowly deteriorates or you can start to do something about it *now*.

So get up!

Whatever you do or dream you can do-begin it.

Boldness has genius and power and magic in it."

-Johann Goethe

Suggested Reading on Nutrition

Nutrition can be a very complicated subject and there are many different points of view on what's healthy and what's not. But there is no doubt that your overall health and wellbeing is directly tied to the foods you consume. It is my belief that to find your own right way to eat, it is important to educate yourself and then find a system that works for you and your personal tastes. Because, let's face it: if you hate the food you eat, you won't eat it for long no matter how good it is for you. I have compiled a list of books that I believe can help you find a healthy way to eat and allow you to choose what best suits your lifestyle and taste. Bon Appétit!

The China Study, By .T Colin Campbell, PhD & Thomas M. Campbell, II

Eat Your Way to Sexy, By Elizabeth Somer, M.A.,R.D.

Real Food, By Nina Planck

What to Eat, By Luise Light, M.S., Ed.D.

Age-Proof Your Body, By Elizabeth Somer, M.A.,R.D.

Staying Healthy with Nutrition, By Elson M. Hass, MD & Buck Levin, PhD, RD

The Paleo Diet, By Loren Cordain, Ph.D

In Defense of Food, By Michael Pollan

Printed in Great Britain
by Amazon

84734547R00102